latent clusters

D1760065

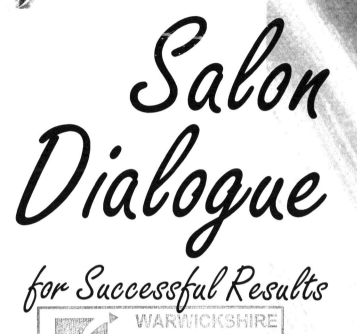

Salon Dialogue

for Successful Results

WARWICKSHIRE COLLEGE LIBRARY

Warwickshire College

00106607

Online Services

Delmar Online
To access a wide variety of Delmar products and services on the World Wide Web,
point your browser to:
>   **http://www.delmar.com**
>   or email: info@delmar.com

thomson.com
To access International Thomson Publishing's
home site for information on more than 34 publishers
and 20,000 products, point your browser to:
>   **http://www.thomson.com**
>   or email: findit@kiosk.thomson.com

A service of I(T)P®

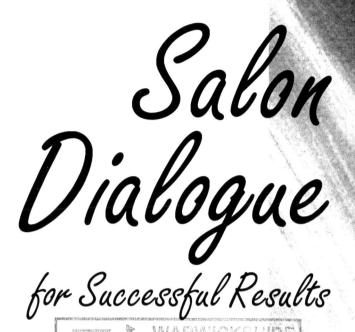

Salon Dialogue

for Successful Results

WARWICKSHIRE COLLEGE LIBRARY

by

Lee Hoffman

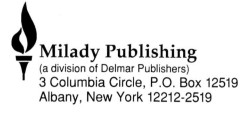

Milady Publishing
(a division of Delmar Publishers)
3 Columbia Circle, P.O. Box 12519
Albany, New York 12212-2519

NOTICE TO THE READER

Publisher does not warrant or guarantee any of the products described herein or perform any independent analysis in connection with any of the product information contained herein. Publisher does not assume, and expressly disclaims, any obligation to obtain and include information other than that provided to it by the manufacturer.

The reader is expressly warned to consider and adopt all safety precautions that might be indicated by the activities herein and to avoid all potential hazards. By following the instructions contained herein, the reader willingly assumes all risks in connections with such instructions.

The publisher makes no representation or warranties of any kind, including but not limited to, the warranties of fitness for particular purpose or merchantability, nor are any such representations implied with respect to the material set forth herein, and the publisher takes no responsibility with respect to such material. The publisher shall not be liable for any special, consequential, or exemplary damages resulting, in whole or part, from the readers' use of, or reliance upon, this material.

Cover Design: Spiral Design Studio

Milady Staff
Publisher: Gordon Miller
Acquisitions Editor: Joseph Miranda
Project Editor: Nancy Jean Downey
Production Manager: Brian Yacur
Art/Design Production Coordinator: Suzanne Nelson

COPYRIGHT © 1998
Milady Publishing
(a division of Delmar Publishers)
an International Thomson Publishing company I(T)P®

£44-99
WARWICKSHIRE COLLEGE
LIBRARY
Class No:
646.72401 HOF
Acc. No:
00106607
Date: Jan '08

Printed in the United States of America
Printed and distributed simultaneously in Canada

For more information, contact:
SalonOvations
Milady Publishing
3 Columbia Circle , Box 12519
Albany, New York   12212-2519

All rights reserved. No part of this work covered by the copyright hereon may be reproduced or used in any form or by any means—graphic, electronic, or mechanical, including photocopying, recording, taping, or information storage and retrieval systems—without the written permission of the publisher.

    4 5 6 7 8 9 10 11 XXX 09 08 07 06

Library of Congress Cataloging-in-Publication Data

Hoffman, Lee.
    Salon dialogue for successful results / by Lee Hoffman.
       p.   cm.
    ISBN: 1-56253-322-3
    1. Beauty operators. 2. Interpersonal communication. I. Milady Publishing Company. II. Title
TT958.H63—8 1997   97-11256
646.7'2'068—dc21   CIP

Contents

8 The Prospective Client   159

9 Consultations   177

Introduction

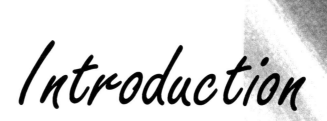

This personal success book is all about how to increase your conversation power.

Some people think that because they are outgoing, they communicate well; however, simply being a person who always has something to say does not qualify them as a conversationalist. No matter how outgoing or how timid you are, achieving conversation power will help you attain success and help avoid many difficult situations.

Conversation power will help you do these things:

Develop strong, long-lasting relationships with clients.

Overcome timidness.

Prevent "foot in mouth" discomfort.

Increase sales and repeat sales.

Avoid disagreements.

Get better information.

Get information faster.

Diffuse anger in others.

Explain more clearly.

Reduce hurt feelings.

Reduce conflicts.

Gain cooperation.

Influence others to your way of thinking.

Develop more supportive relationships.

When you work as a service professional, success depends on how well you communicate with others. To be successful in your professional life, you must communicate with co-workers, clients, prospective clients, and your boss; and to be successful in your personal life, you must have effective communication with family, friends, and community.

The difference between service professionals who earn high incomes and those who settle for low incomes is simply sales. Without sales and repeat sales, there is no income. From the first conversation on the phone, continuing through the service and the client checkout, every word exchanged between the client and salon staff is critical to the success of the sale.

There are multitudes of stylists who say they are not sales-people, but they spend all day selling to customers. Recently a stylist at Sensations Salon was overheard saying to her client, "Did you see the movie *The Twist of Fate*? It was really great. It kept me on the edge of my seat for the entire movie. It's playing at the new theater in town. Have you been there yet? It's a great place—ten theaters—it's clean and they have popcorn done with that good oil. . . ." Instead of selling shampoo, conditioner, or services to the client, she was selling the movie, the theater, and the popcorn.

Too often salon professionals sell clothes for their favorite specialty stores, CDs, great restaurants, etc. They sell everything that they like except salon services and products. Perhaps one reason this happens is that stylists don't know how to approach clients about product sales and services.

For many years, professionals in the cosmetology industry have focused on learning listening skills. In fact, their education has been so one sided in favor of listening that when the conversation dies between salon professionals and clients, stylists don't know how to revive it. Both clients and stylists search for something to fill the void. Since it's human nature to talk about themselves, when there's nothing left to say, that is the conversation topic they're most comfortable with. For example, clients may ask "How was your weekend?" That small nudge from clients is all most stylists need to begin expounding the wonders of the latest dance bar to open downtown, their children's accomplishments, or their latest surgery. Often, the salon professional never returns to the realm of the client again.

The best salespeople in the world know the words, the questions, and the feedback that lead a conversation where they want it to go—toward sales. It is much easier to lead a client if you know exactly what to say and how to say it and especially if you have a procedure for it.

Salon dialogue is the procedure that tells you how to lead conversations with clients that result in better sales and higher client retention rates. Some salon dialogues are specific word-by-word scripts. Others are guidelines for communicating, and still others are strategies for scripts in specific situations.

As you read and learn about salon dialogue, you will get to know the staff of Sensations Salon as they communicate with their clients and each other. Important concept dialogues are indicated throughout the book by using caricatures of the Sensations staff.

You will discover how to create sales scripts by learning the substructure of communication, which consists of body language, voice, and words. Then you will learn about the foundation of communication, which includes learning about different types of clients, and you will master the structure of the script itself.

In later chapters, you will learn how the Sensations staff uses conversation power to develop rapport with clients on the phone, attract prospective clients, and smooth out difficult situations. You will experience their failures at communicating as well as their successes at working with customers in everyday situations. Perhaps you will be familiar with some of the problems and circumstances.

Communication Power

*T*oday at the Sensations Salon, Janet, a stylist, has asked Carl, the color technician, for advice about an upcoming competition. Janet wants to know whether or not she should color her model's hair.

Janet: *Carl, this is my friend Isatou. Remember, she is the one I'm using for the competition next month.*

Carl: *Nice to meet you. Your name is I . . .?*

Isatou: *Isatou. I . . . Sa . . . Tu.*

Carl: *Isatou. That is a beautiful name.*

Isatou: *Thank you, Carl. I'm happy to meet you, too.*

Janet: *Carl, what I need is some color advice. Do you think I should add more red to Isatou's hair, or would I be better off just putting a glaze on it for shine?*

Isatou: *Janet, remember, I've never had my hair tinted before. I don't know if I would like red.*

Carl: *Isatou, you have beautiful hair and skin. You would look great in red as long as it was more mahogany than auburn. Look at the hair color in this photograph.* (Carl shows Isatou a photo from an album.) *That's the color you should wear. And we have another option. I think we could use a semipermanent color rather than a permanent one on you. How does that sound?*

Isatou: *That sounds better. That means that it would wash out, right?*

Carl: *Yes, it would eventually wash out. Now, what is the style going to look like, Janet?*

Janet: *Well, the front will have an asymmetric wave, the sides will be flat and smooth, and I'm integrating a hairpiece into the back.*

Carl: *What is the focus of the style?*

Janet: *Focus?*

Carl: *This is your first competition, isn't it?*

Janet: *Yes, it is my first time, and it's getting more involved than I thought. I don't know if I really want to do it.*

Carl: *You're getting a little scared, aren't you? Janet, you are a fantastic hairdresser and I know you'll do a great job in the competition. Now mock up that style for me so I can find the focal point.*

Janet: *Thanks, Carl.*

> *Communication is trading information so that all parties understand the subject matter in the same way.*

Communication Power

True communication involves speaking, listening, and giving feedback. Communication is trading information so that all parties understand the subject matter in the same way. When genuine communication exists, everybody sees the same picture.

We already know that if we don't listen to our clients, they will find another salon professional who will hear their needs. During the past decade, we have learned much about listening but very little about the other half of communication—speaking.

The speaking part of communication is just as important as the listening side. You can listen all day to clients talk, but does that bring sales, create success, or give you any future security? No, it doesn't. When you listen, you are receiving and processing information. When you speak, you give and clarify the information.

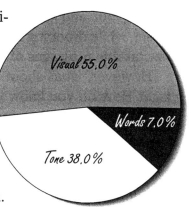

Research shows that in communication you give and receive information in three ways. Visual communication accounts for 55% of the message and is the way you express yourself through body language. Communication through tone, which is 38% of the information, refers to your voice; and finally, communication through data, the specific words you use, accounts for only 7%.

Body Language

Body language is the way we express ourselves with our body movements, such as our posture, gestures, and facial expressions. It is as important to understand our clients' body language as it is to be aware of the message that we convey to our clients through our own body language.

We use the term *meta-message* to describe those messages that come between the lines; they come from the relationship, the timing, the purpose, and the person speaking. For example, Susan calls her friend Dave for the third time in one day. She says, "Hi, it's me again." He responds, "I'm working on this photo layout, and it's due in half an hour." His message is not intended as an update on his progress. His words and tone mean, "Why are you bothering me again? I haven't time to talk now."

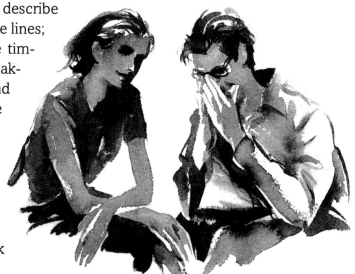

Certain body language is easy to read. Hands on hips,

a tapping foot, and looking at a watch are all obvious signs of discontent, while drooping shoulders, giant sighs, and sad looks are unmistakable messages of depression.

However, what about the more subtle forms of body language? How do you know if a client trusts you? What does her body say when she is comfortable with you? How would her facial expression tell you she is unhappy with the way her nails look?

Consider the messages you unknowingly convey to your client:

- A tiring colorist leans heavily on the styling chair, looking drained and exhausted. He moves slowly, like a "dying warrior," and needs only a drooping feather across his brow to complete the sad picture. Imagine how his client feels.
- The "walkie talkie" nail tech is never quiet or still for even a moment. Perhaps her actions are screaming insecurity to her client.
- The impatient stylist shuffles in one spot, sometimes even cracking knuckles as he waits like a "chained elephant" for the client to move along, choose a new style, or decide on a color.
- The "flittering bird" body language of a new haircutter, who jumps from one spot to another while cutting or uses her hands with stiff jerky movements, may be showing incompetence to her client.
- The "swordsman" talks with his comb or, worse yet, his haircutting shears. His client wonders if he knows where he left off in the haircut.

If you would like to hone your body language skills, the chart should help.

Reading Faces

Important information is disclosed through facial expressions. When you are angry, it is difficult to prevent your lips from narrowing; it happens even before you realize the anger. Be aware of facial expressions while working in the salon, where there are

Body Language Messages

Message	Posture	Facial Expression
Caregiving	Leaning forward Rounded shoulders Arm around another's shoulders	Pity Bent head
Open	Straight, smooth Loose, calm Few gestures	Relaxed Eye contact Neutral
Offensive	Stiff Chin out Arms across chest	Flashing eyes Teeth bared Clenched teeth
Controlling Angry	Tense shoulders Hands on hips Arms folded Shaking head	Pursed lips Glaring Rolling eyes Grim looks
Spontaneous	Relaxed Fluid Touching	Smiling Wide eyed

mirrors everywhere. A client could see confusion or disdain by the way you move your lips and eyebrows.

Clients' facial expressions convey information, too. A young client might convey fear by a slight lifting and pulling together of the eyebrows and a widening of the eyes. Faces are easy to read on children because they haven't learned that society frowns on open display of emotions. As people mature they learn the rules of emotional display that tell them where and when they can safely express their feelings. Adults learn not to show disappointment; therefore, they seldom cry in public—unless, of course, the tears are joyful, as when loved ones are reunited.

Simply watching a person's eyebrows can give you many conversational clues. Raising one eyebrow is a strong indication that your listener is doubtful or a little surprised by what he or she has heard. To emphasize a phrase, people will usually raise or lower their eyebrows. Joining together of the eyebrows indicates that the listener is thinking or puzzled. When you see that

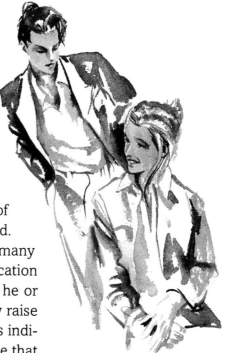

expression on your client, it means you should clarify your statement.

Often stylists communicate between themselves by using facial expressions. You may use facial expressions to order lunch confidentially from a co-worker who is making a trip to pickup take-out food; however, your client could be offended by the message she interprets from your expressions which she sees in the mirror. If this happens during a client's chemical service the client could fear that something had gone wrong and the stylist was summoning help. Additionally, an insecure first time client might see this form of communication as rude.

Lips and mouths also convey many different messages. Lips can create a variety of frowns as well as a medley of smiles; they can disclose emotions from despair to joy. You can recognize a smile of enjoyment by the crinkling of the small muscles around the eyes. A polite social smile is often tilted more on one side than the other, and it usually involves only the lip muscles. A grin-and-bear-it smile is the one your client might display when you say that her hair really must be permed to get the style she wants. She might not like getting a perm, but she'll go along with it to get the results she wants.

Tone and Voice

Your voice, used as tone, accounts for 38% of the information you give and receive. To get a message across to listeners, we make use of many elements in addition to body language. Besides shrugging our shoulders, moving our arms, and wrinkling our brows, we can increase the volume and vary the pitch and the pace of our voice. We change the inflection of our voice and talk rapidly or slowly as the occasion and the material may dictate.

Tone and quality of voice have little to do with the words we use. Think about how babies communicate. A mother knows by the sound of the cry whether her baby is sleepy, hungry, needs to be changed, or just wants to be held. We use our voice tone and quality to express emotions, to command attention, and to make a point. Words are powerless without tone.

Most of us lose spontaneity and naturalness of tone as we grow older. With age, we tend to slip into a definite mold of physical and vocal communication. We find ourselves less animated and less emotional in our speech, and we rarely raise or lower our voices from one pitch to another.

Success in the salon business depends on one-to-one communication, so it is important that we use varying voice tones and inflections. Your voice can reflect your intelligence and professionalism or lack of it. It exposes your attitude and your emotions. And it can be trained to be the kind of voice you want it to be.

Qualities of Voice

Pitch   The pitch of your voice can be high or low. Speech experts say that low is desirable because it projects and carries better; it is also more pleasant. Through practice, you can cultivate a rich, sonorous voice.

Inflection   Your voice inflection shows your emotions and makes you a more interesting person to talk to. A voice without inflection is monotone and leaves the listener clueless about the speaker's true feelings. Rising inflection toward the end of a sentence leaves the listener anticipating the next sentence. Imagine a sentence such as "There is a fire in this building" spoken without inflection of any kind. Would you know if the speaker meant a fire in a fireplace or a dangerous fire requiring emergency action? Imagine if the same sentence was screamed, "There's a fire in this building!" You would have no doubt about the meaning.

Courtesy   Common everyday courtesy is most important in a service business, especially when you are on the phone and you can't see the person to whom you are speaking. A courteous voice should be pleasant and reflect patience and caring.

Loudness   Loud and soft tones also reveal emotions. Often it isn't what you say but how you say it. The loudness of your voice can reflect sincerity, confidence, and interest as well as anger and impatience.

Understandability   Avoid talking with anything in your mouth (chewing gum, pencils, etc.). Don't mumble. If you have a southern drawl or any other regional accent, don't think you have to change it. Accents, as long as the words are easily understood, make you a unique and memorable person.

Success in the salon business depends on one-to-one communication, so it is important that we use varying voice tones and inflections.

Rate The basic rate of speech is 140 words per minute (wpm). If you speak too rapidly, people start listening to how fast you're talking instead of what you are saying. Speaking too slowly can be irritating to listeners because they are kept hanging on every word, and they tend to anticipate what you are going to say next.

Enunciation Carefully enunciate your words. Keep your T's and D's straight as well as your F's and X's. While crisp clear enunciation declares that you mean business, sloppy "words" like "umgonna," "I gotta," or "wud ya think" might make your client think you are as careless about your work as you are about your speech.

The most interesting voices vary loud and soft and know when to use silence instead of a filler sound such as "uh."

Avoid patronizing, condescending, or egotistic voice tones. A patronizing person always expresses an opinion and makes those with expertise feel stupid for having such expertise. People have a strong urge to argue with a patronizing individual, even if they don't really disagree.

If you are condescending to clients, they will feel that you won't say what you really think and therefore you are untrustworthy. If a client can't trust you, he will not buy from you.

Use professional vocabulary. Because your grammar and vocabulary reveal your level of education, slang and vulgarism, no matter how common or popular, do not belong in the vocabulary you use at work.

Analyzing Your Voice

Recording your voice on a tape recorder is a great way to listen for voice quality and irritating vocal habits. Frequent use of "uh," "OK," or "ya know what I mean" between phrases is a signature of an undisciplined voice. The most pleasant voices use various pitches and avoid monotones. The most interesting voices also vary loud and soft and know when to use silence instead of a filler sound such as "uh."

You can practice voice tones by doing the following activity. Record yourself on tape or practice with a friend. Express the emotions happy, sad, angry, and afraid with each of the following sentences. Observe how the meaning changes with the different emotions.

1. I'm sorry.

2. Where did you get that information?

3. I don't know.

4. When will it be ready?

5. Here, let me help.

6. Is there something I can do?

7. Mr. Smith will take care of that.

8. I forgot.

9. I made a mistake.

10. I'm busy.

11. I'm not able to do that.

12. That's true.

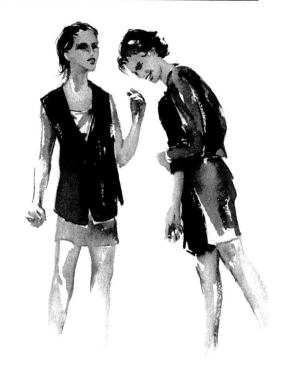

Words

Even though only 7% of the information you give or receive is in the form of spoken words, don't discount them. Words make conversation more specific. There are words that work overtime for us and others that we should forget.

We use words to control other people's actions. The words we choose in any given situation can either turn a client away or create a long-lasting client/stylist relationship.

Here are some scripts that turn clients off:

Did I cut your hair like this?

I would be really upset if my hair was ruined like yours.

I can't do anything with your hair unless you get a perm.

Your hair is so flat and lifeless, how do you live with it?

This hairstyle is really outdated.

You are really having a bad hair day.

Some phrases cut off options for your client. On the other hand, some expressions guide your client to better alternatives.

Avoid: *You have to . . . You can't . . .*

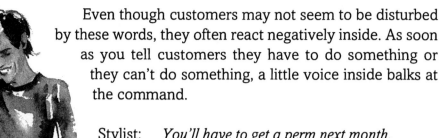

Even though customers may not seem to be disturbed by these words, they often react negatively inside. As soon as you tell customers they have to do something or they can't do something, a little voice inside balks at the command.

Stylist: *You'll have to get a perm next month.*

Client's thought: *I don't have to do anything.*

Instead use: *Will you . . . Can you . . . Would you like to . . .*

Example: *Your perm is starting to grow out. Would you like to schedule a perm next month so that your style stays looking good?*

Avoid: *Why don't you . . .*

Did you ever ask a small child 'Why?" The answer is always "because." Sometimes our suggestions work; however, you have probably encountered a client who finds all the reasons why something you suggest won't work. When you say to a client, "Why don't you get a pedicure with your manicure next time?" your client's mind will focus on why she shouldn't, rather than the benefits of having the service.

Instead use: *Have you considered . . . It works great to . . .*

Example: *Have you considered getting a pedicure with your manicure? Wouldn't it be nice to have your feet looking beautiful to go on your vacation? It works great to schedule them together. That way you don't have to spend any more time here.*

Avoid: *It's not our policy . . .*

This common phrase is a way of hiding from confrontation.

Example: *It is salon policy that all clients change into a client gown before any chemical services.*

When it really is or isn't your salon policy, simply state the reasons for the policy rather than reciting the policy itself.

Instead use: *The reasons why . . .*

Example: *Please change into this gown. We want to be sure that your clothing doesn't get damaged from solutions during color or perming. Just one drop could ruin your beautiful sweater.*

Avoid: *I'll try . . .*

Client: *I don't like the way that other stylist cut my son's hair. It isn't short enough in the back, and the front is uneven. I know he likes her to cut his hair, but it's awful. Can you do something about it?*

Stylist: *Sure, I'll try to do something.*

When you say you'll try, you surrender your power and responsibility, and your client is left hanging. When you don't give a client closure on an issue or problem, you relinquish the client's trust.

Sometimes our suggestions work; however, you have probably encountered a client who finds all the reasons why something you suggest won't work.

Instead use: *This is what I can do . . . I can do this . . .*

Example: *I will talk to the manager about giving you a credit on it. Would you like me to recut it, or would you prefer that his regular stylist redo it?*

Avoid: *But . . .*

The use of *but* after a statement negates everything that was said before.

Stylist: *I understand that you aren't happy with your perm and you need it redone, but your stylist is on vacation.*

Instead use: *However . . . and . . .*

Example: *I understand that you aren't happy with your perm and since your stylist is on vacation, we can schedule with another stylist or you can wait till next week when she comes back.*

When you substitute *however* or *and*, you will provide smooth transition to new information, options, or alternatives.

| **Avoid:** | *The best thing . . . The worst thing . . .* |
| Stylist: | *The best thing you could do is invest in conditioning treatments for those damaged ends.* |

Often, telling a client "The best thing" or "The worst thing" makes you seem like you are making judgments and cutting off options for your client.

| Instead use: | *It would work well to . . . What would happen if . . .* |
| Example: | *It would work well to have a series of conditioning treatments on those ends. Or, what would happen if you got some of the worst split ends trimmed?* |

The most powerful word you can use is your client's name. Everyone wants to be recognized. Even for people who seem indifferent, the deepest cut of all is to be ignored. Call your clients by their correct names. Mangling or mispronouncing a client's name can lose the client. Our name is the only thing we can exclusively call our own. It distinguishes us from others and makes us feel important.

For example, Margaret might get angry if you call her Peg or Margie, and so might Robert if you call him Bob or Bobby when he wants to be called Robert. Consider also the client who, rather than her first name Elizabeth, chooses to be called Mrs. Jones.

Remembering your client's name is easy when it's right in front of you on the appointment book, the client questionnaire, and the client file. To make it a more permanent part of your memory, practice using the name during the consultation and write it down when you make notes in the client file.

Fifty Emotion-Packed Words

Some words almost automatically have a strong emotional appeal no matter how they are used. Communication experts have singled out these power-laden words, and the research of those experts has proved valuable to salespeople and to anyone trying to influence other people.

How many of these words can you tie to your products and services?

1. Scientific	18. Health	35. Discovery
2. New	19. Quality	36. Patriotism
3. Clean	20. Elegance	37. Recommended
4. Efficient	21. Bargain	38. Sociable
5. Timesaving	22. Sympathy	39. Stylish
6. Appetizing	23. Trend	40. Royalty
7. Value	24. Courtesy	41. Admired
8. Affectionate	25. Growth	42. Beauty
9. Fun	26. Amusement	43. Personality
10. Ambition	27. Hospitality	44. Independent
11. Reputation	28. Status	45. Successful
12. Guaranteed	29. Enormous	46. Up-to-date
13. Stimulating	30. Low-cost	47. Tested
14. Safe	31. Genuine	48. Expressive
15. Popular	32. Progress	49. Relief
16. Economical	33. Thinking	50. Tasteful
17. Modern	34. Excel	

The most powerful word you can use is your client's name. Everyone wants to be recognized.

To categorize these power words, we can separate them according to age groups. If you want to attract clients over age sixty, use any words that relate to value, such as word 21, *bargain*, or word 12, *guaranteed*.

To attract more clients in the age group forty to sixty, use words that relate to being healthy, like word 3, *clean*, and word 14, *safe*.

For clients in the age bracket of twenty-five to forty, the key words are *looking good* and *success*. Words 15, *popular*, 28, *status*, and 25, *growth*, would be power words for this age group. To attract clients under age twenty-five, use word 6, *appetizing*, word 13, *stimulating*, word 39, *stylish*, or word 26, *amusement*. People under age twenty-five tend to buy something just because it appeals to them.

More Scripts to Avoid and Scripts to Learn

Stylist: *I don't know.*

Replace with: *That's a good question, I'll find out for you.*

Stylist:	We can't do that.
Replace with:	This is what we can do. Or, next time this happens, this is what you can do.
Stylist:	Hang on a second.
Replace with:	I need a few minutes to check on your request; do you mind if I put you on hold? or, can you hold for just a minute, or, would you prefer that I call you back?
Stylist:	No.
Replace with:	Let's see what we can do.

Caring Responses

Build rapport with clients by using caring responses. When customer service lacks caring and friendliness, it also lacks the qualities that encourage loyalty in a customer. The objective in customer service is for the client to leave the salon feeling well cared for and wanting to come back again. By using simple caring responses during conversations with clients, you will achieve that goal.

Acknowledging clients happens in two ways: first, when you greet clients, and second, during your conversations with them. When a client mentions a vacation, a child's achievements, or a new job, you can quickly acknowledge the comment with responses such as these:

That's great!
Terrific!
Wonderful!
You don't say!

If clients tell you personal facts, they do so because they want acknowledgment. Not responding can make clients feel that you are ignoring them. In return, they can become angry or embarrassed at your lack of caring.

When clients demonstrate concern, acknowledge their feelings by being empathetic to their situation. If you use an apology, be sure to include a reason.

I'm sorry to hear that your mother has been ill.
I'm sorry that you're having difficulty with your new haircut.

If clients have a concern that is directed at your performance or at the salon, assure them that you will be responsible for taking care of it.

I will take care of that for you.
I'll check with Margo about it as soon as I finish your hair.

Appreciating clients, another caring response, doesn't have to wait until the client is leaving the salon. You can appreciate something about a client at any time during their visit.

Thanks for your patience. I'm sorry you had to wait so long.
I really enjoy cutting your hair!
I'm glad you are my client.
I really appreciate . . . (your referrals, your business, your loyalty, your willingness to try new styles, etc.).

When you end a service with a client, use an extended thank you.

Thank you (client's name), I enjoyed working with you today.
Thanks for coming in (client's name), I really appreciate your business.

Sincere compliments are also caring responses. Be sure that the compliment is authentic and doesn't sound manufactured.

I love your jacket.
I love working with hair like yours.
You have beautiful skin.

The objective in customer service is for the client to leave the salon feeling well cared for and wanting to come back again.

Customers perceive caring responses as a demonstration of their importance to you. Friendly gestures create rapport with clients, while a lack of caring responses is perceived as cold and detached.

Mindful Listening

The most misunderstood communication skill is listening. Many people equate silence with listening, and nothing could be further from the truth. Listening requires active thinking, body language, and feeling; while silence is nothing more than keeping your mouth shut. Mindful listening means absorbing the content of what you are hearing from the speaker.

Poor listeners forget names and details. The more you use a client's name and repeat the main details of the client's life, the easier it will be to remember such things. Ideally, taking notes while consulting with your client is the best way to keep track of your client today and in the future.

Carla is a first-time client. Her stylist today is Marc. By the time he has introduced himself, given Carla a tour of the salon, and finished the basic consultation, he has already used Carla's name six times, referred to her home town of Albany twice, and learned the ages of her three children. Some of his questions and comments were as follows:

Marc: *Carla, did you have your hair done in downtown Albany or nearer your home in the suburbs?*

Carla: *Downtown. It was more convenient to go to a salon near my office. I could have my color, haircut, or nails done during my lunch break. That way I didn't have to take time from my kids in the evenings or on Saturdays.*

Marc: *I bet you really like living here, where your work is just a few minutes from home.*

Carla: *It is nice to know I'm always close to my kids now.*

Marc: *I like your cut. Have you been wearing it for a long time? It would also look good with the back a little shorter. What do you think, Carla?*

Mindful listening requires looking for hidden communication clues (this is sometimes called reading between the lines or reading the hidden message).

Client Barbara: *I don't know what to do about my haircolor. It just doesn't match my skin tone since I got back from vacation. Even my lipstick doesn't work. Do you see how tan I am?*

Stylist Jennifer: *I think the color we have been doing is lovely. Maybe you should get a conditioning treatment to counteract the effects of the sun.*

Barbara: *It's the color I'm concerned about. It just doesn't seem to go with my tan. I don't know what to do. I've never had a tan this time of year before.*

Jennifer: *I don't think you should change your haircolor just because you have a tan. Besides, in a few weeks you'll be pale again. Let's just stick with the old color and do a conditioning treatment.*

Barbara: *I like my tan and I just might keep it. Do you have any ideas?*

The most misunderstood communication skill is listening. Many people equate silence with listening, and nothing could be further from the truth.

Good listeners almost never miss a conversational clue. Tune into the whole person for these hidden messages, not just the words. Obviously, Jennifer didn't hear the unspoken words that her client, Barbara, had just returned from a vacation and was looking for a compliment on her great tan.

Listening Barriers

There are many obstacles that prevent us from listening as actively as we should. The primary barrier is daydreaming. We daydream because we have more time mentally than we need. We talk about 140 words per minute but listen at a speedy 400 words per minute. There is too much time to think between the speaker's words. It's easy to start thinking about what to say next, about a popular movie you are seeing tonight, or about the color problem you are having with your next client.

The second common barrier is surroundings. Too much noise and too many disruptions will distract you from your client. Blow dryers can be so loud that your client will feel the need to shout over the noise made at the next station. Salon music can be distracting and sometimes irritating. It's a good rule to play music that your clients like instead of the music the staff enjoys. Background music in the salon should be barely loud enough to hear the words. Loud staff members can be irritating as well as distracting. Just because some people naturally have loud voices doesn't mean they can't quiet down—it just takes some practice.

Selective listening is the third barrier to attentiveness. We begin listening selectively because we think we already know what the client is going to say next. Sometimes we prejudge the speaker instead of listening to find out what we don't know. Did you ever balk at having a refresher product knowledge class because you already "know" the product only to discover that you didn't know many little tidbits about it?

Interrupting is the fourth barrier to good listening. There is nothing worse than a listener who interrupts the speaker continually. Interrupting is the most obvious way of saying to the speaker, "I'm important and you are not."

Interruptions occur in many ways, such as when you must take a phone call, when another staff member must ask a question, even when another client breaks in to say "Hi." Avoid interruptions whenever possible. Don't take phone calls unless it's an emergency, ask other staff members to avoid disturbing you when you're with a client, and ask them to respect the space you need for your client.

Another frequent type of interruption occurs when a stylist must leave to check on another client. It may be impossible to eliminate interruptions, but it is conceivable to reduce the number of disruptions. When you must leave your client, always apologize and ask to be excused. When you return, thank the client for his or her patience, take a minute to recenter yourself, review what you have done, and then resume your work.

Marc: *Excuse me, Betty, I have to leave you for just a minute to check a perm that is processing.*

Betty: *Sure, Marc, go ahead.*

Marc (*when he returns*):   *Thank you for waiting, Betty. OK, now let me see where I left off.*

Imagine you are a client getting a haircut. Your stylist leaves quickly, runs back, picks up shears, and immediately begins to cut. Would you wonder if that stylist was thinking about your haircut or the perm that is processing? Recentering on clients is a way of reassuring them that you are in control and that they are your top priority. Before you resume cutting, simply take a few seconds to review the work you have already done.

The final obstacle, not being prepared for your client, is the easiest to overcome. Being prepared means preparing mentally as well as physically. It's hard to listen to a client while you are cleaning up from the last client. It is equally hard to concentrate on a client if your mind is thinking about the color client you did earlier today or what you are wearing to dinner tonight. Using a client questionnaire or client information sheet and a client file system will help you be mentally prepared to listen to your client.

Listening barriers include daydreaming, distracting surroundings, selective listening, interruptions, and not being prepared for your client.

Reflective Listening

In reflective listening, you feed back to the customer what his or her feelings seem to be. You're not participating in the customer's point of view, just commenting on it. Reflective listening will help you keep your attention focused on your customer's emotions. For example, when a customer says, "I just don't know if I should get my hair tinted," your reflection is, "It sounds like you're apprehensive about getting your hair colored."

Paraphrasing

To paraphrase or give feedback is to restate your client's words to be sure you heard correctly. Rewording, interpreting, and summarizing are also forms of paraphrasing. For example, when a customer says, "I've talked to two technicians about my nails, done everything they said to do, and they are still breaking!"—your paraphrase is, "You say you've talked to two people already and no one has helped you?"

Nonverbal Listening Cues

Eye Contact

Eye contact is so powerful in our culture that we can beckon for a co-worker's help, invite a lover, or even summon a taxi driver by "catching" that person's eye. The eyes, it is said, are the mirrors of the soul. It is no wonder that a person who doesn't look you in the eye is thought to be untrustworthy. Eyes usually convey a nonverbal message consistent with spoken words. When there is an inconsistency, truth will show in the eyes. If a client says she is "Just fine" but her eyes are sad and sorrowful, which message do you believe?

Maintaining eye contact with clients lets them know that you are paying attention. However, be careful not to stare or maintain the contact after the client has broken contact. Continuing to stare could be considered impolite or even disrespectful.

Eyes usually convey a nonverbal message consistent with spoken words. . . The way we touch or refrain from touching people communicates much about our personalities.

Touching

The way we touch or refrain from touching people communicates much about our personalities. Clients know by the way we touch them if we are confident, insecure, timid, or extroverted. A new cosmetology student might express how insecure he is by the way he shampoos a client, or a tense haircutter will convey his nervousness by the way he combs his client's hair and touches his client's head. A positive, reassuring touch will tell a client that you are listening and are empathetic to her situation.

In many industries, pats, squeezes, brushes, and hugs become the basis of sexual harassment charges. Although our industry isn't immune to such charges, sexual harassment is less likely to happen between clients and stylists or technicians. Fortunately, salon professionals are expected to touch their clients. Therefore, it is much easier for clients to accept a steadying hand on the arm, a pat on the back, or a hand on the shoulder.

Smiling

There is no better way to build rapport with clients than greeting them with a sincere smile. A genuine smile shows on the rest of your face—in the lines around your eyes, cheeks, and forehead.

Be careful about using a fake smile. When a person has a perpetual smile on his or her face, we might wonder if that person is a politician, is dishonest, or is a sly salesman. It is obvious when a smile is patronizing, or when it shows nervousness or even pain. Learn to smile only to show amusement or express genuine emotions.

Nodding

Did you ever talk to someone and feel like you were talking to a wall? Perhaps the other party was listening but was not giving you any nonverbal cues. Nodding is an excellent tool to show someone you are listening to him or her. It can say, "Yes, I hear you." It can also signify agreement or empathy, depending on the situation.

Spacing

Did you ever notice that in an interesting conversation the participants will lean forward and sometimes even move toward the speaker? The amount of personal space a person needs changes according to circumstances. The closer the relationship, the less space is needed. In a business atmosphere, 4 to 12 feet is an acceptable space for conversing. In a private conversation, personal space can be as little as 1 foot.

To show a client you are listening, lean slightly toward the client. If you are a stylist, occasionally walk around the client and speak to him or her face to face rather than through the mirror.

Mirroring Energy

To mirror energy, observe whether clients move calmly and smoothly or if their movements are quick and precise; then match your energy level to your client. Note whether a client's mood is happy, sad, joyful, reflective, etc., and try to get into a corresponding mood. It isn't necessary for you to become sad because a client is sad; however, you should be receptive to that client's need to be sad.

Chapter Summary

1. What you say and how you say it have a significant impact on your success as a salon professional.
2. Specific scripted sentences for each salon situation will guide you toward being an excellent communicator.
3. True communication combines speaking and feedback with active listening.
4. Body language is visual communication. Learning to read body language is imperative in effective communication.
5. The tone and quality of your voice accounts for 38% of your communication to clients.
6. Good voice quality can be learned. Analyze your own voice by using a recorder.
7. Voice inflection and loudness show emotion.
8. 7% of the information you give or receive is in the form of spoken words. Words make conversation more specific, add color, and spark interest in a conversation.
9. If you want to attract clients over age sixty, use any words

that relate to "value," such as *bargain* or *guaranteed*. To attract more clients in the age group forty to sixty, use words that relate to healthy, like *clean* and *safe*. For clients in the age bracket twenty-five to forty, the key words are *looking good* and *success*. *Popular, status*, and *growth* would be a few power words for this age group. To attract clients under age twenty-five, use words like *appetizing, stimulation, stylish*, or *amusement*, because people in that age group tend to buy more just because it appeals to them.

10. Build rapport with clients by using caring responses. The objective in customer service is for the client to leave the salon feeling well cared for and wanting to come back again. By using simple caring responses during conversations with clients, you will achieve that goal.

11. Listening, which is the key communication skill, requires active thinking, body language, and feeling. Active listening means absorbing the content of what you are hearing from the speaker.

12. Mindful listening requires looking for hidden communication clues in conversations.

13. Barriers to listening are daydreaming, prejudging what the other person is saying, interrupting, and being in distracting surroundings.

14. Reflective listening, paraphrasing, and giving feedback are all communication skills that clarify a conversation. Reflective listening reflects the client's feelings, paraphrasing repeats the client's words in another way, and feedback restates the idea in the listener's words.

Scripting a Sale

Margo: *Good morning, Sensations Salon. This is Margo. How may I help you?*

Gloria: *Yes, I have and appointment tomorrow at 5:30 with Monique. I need to cancel it.*

Margo: *You must be Gloria. Is that right?*

Gloria: *Yes. Gloria Heath.*

Margo: *OK. Gloria, I can do that for you. You were scheduled for a color touch-up and haircut, correct?*

Gloria: *Yes, that's right.*

Margo: *I'm sure you don't want to wait too long for your color. How about scheduling a week from now at the same time?*

Gloria: *You're probably right. I always wait and call too late. Go ahead and schedule it.*

Margo: *Great, Gloria, I'll put you down for color and a haircut. Would you like to have a manicure while your color is processing?*

Gloria: *I've never had a manicure.*

Margo: *It's wonderful, Gloria, and it wouldn't take any extra time.*

What you say and how you say it have a significant impact on your professional growth. Few people have that naturally fluid tongue that provides exactly the right words at exactly the right time. For the rest of us, developing that talent requires learning the skills of conversation, such as voice tone, body language, and choice of the best words. Conversation skills pay off handsomely in increased abilities to persuade and motivate your clients. Such skills can be mastered easily by preparing scripts of specific sentences for specific situations. Once you learn the scripts, it becomes easy to be a great conversationalist.

The Benefits of Salon Scripts

Did you ever work with a stylist who looks at the appointment book at the beginning of the day and plans how to sell additional services to existing clients to fill in the empty spaces in the day's schedule? She knows that even adding a brow arch to every client in a day could add as much as 20% to her daily total. But how do you convince a client without sounding like a hard sell? A salon script helps you do so in a way that will lead a client to thank you for taking the time do all those little things for her that other stylists neglected.

Add-On Services

Salon scripts teach you how to detect the services that even the client didn't know she needed and suggest add-on services to your client (resulting in higher daily tickets).

Nail tech Carolyn: *Good morning, Mrs. White. It's nice to see you again. Let me take a look at your hands before we get started. Has all this cold weather been making your hands feel rough and dry?*

Mrs. White: *It certainly has, and I have been doing so much cleaning lately that my fingertips are beginning to crack. I'm getting ready for my daughter's engagement party tomorrow night.*

Carolyn (examines Mrs. White's nails): *You must be really excited about your daughter's engagement! You're having the party at your home?*

Mrs. White: *Yes. I have a large home, and we like to entertain. We have room for fifty as long as I don't try to have a sit-down dinner. Delights Caterers is handling it for me. Do you know them?*

Carolyn (begins the manicure): *I've heard great things about them, Mrs. White. As I look at your hands, I do see how the tips are dry and overworked. I can do an herbology treatment on your hands today that will make them feel like baby's skin. Wouldn't it be nice to have your hands feel good tomorrow with all the hand shaking you'll be doing?*

Mrs. White: *It certainly would. How much is the treatment and how long does it take? I still have a lot of things to do.*

Carolyn: *It's only ten dollars, and it only takes ten minutes longer than your regular manicure. Your hands will thank you for it.*

Mrs. White: *OK. Let's do it.*

Barbara Salomone

Bioelements / Conservatory of Esthetics

Des Plaines, IL

Bioelements suggests recommending additional services to clients. Beside the phone, have a list of recommended companion services that complement each service. This way the receptionist can suggest those services and the client doesn't have to think about it. For example, suggest makeup application after a facial or reflexology with a pedicure or a scalp massage with a haircut.

Establishing Trust

Using salon scripts helps establish trust between the salon professional and the client.

Susan: *Marc, I think I would like to get rid of this gray hair, but I've never put anything on my hair before and I just don't know what would be the best thing to do, or if I should do anything at all.*

Marc: *Susan, you have just a little gray showing at your temples. There are a variety of color services that would work for you. Let me explain them to you, and then we will discuss the advantages of each before you decide which service is right for you.*

Susan: *No one has ever taken the time to explain haircolor to me before.*

Reassuring, confident responses convey competence and professionalism. When a client knows that you understand her needs, she will trust you more. Look at the situation from your own perspective. Would you patronize a business that made you feel uncomfortable? Would you leave your expensive diamond ring with a jeweler if you didn't trust him?

Increasing Client Awareness

Scripting increases the awareness of your available services. Imagine what would happen if you reviewed your salon brochure with every client to make them aware of all the services your salon offers. Look at it from your client's point of view—don't they deserve to know what your salon offers? Imagine if your waiter at a choice restaurant neglected to inform you that your favorite meal was the special of the day. Wouldn't you feel cheated?

John : *Hello, Sandy. How are you today?*

Sandy: *Just great, John. I'm really looking forward to this haircut.*

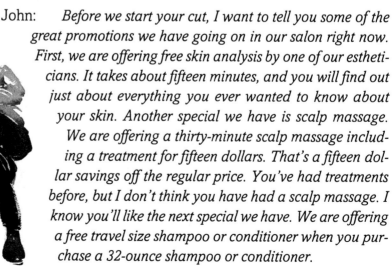

John: *Before we start your cut, I want to tell you some of the great promotions we have going on in our salon right now. First, we are offering free skin analysis by one of our estheticians. It takes about fifteen minutes, and you will find out just about everything you ever wanted to know about your skin. Another special we have is scalp massage. We are offering a thirty-minute scalp massage including a treatment for fifteen dollars. That's a fifteen dollar savings off the regular price. You've had treatments before, but I don't think you have had a scalp massage. I know you'll like the next special we have. We are offering a free travel size shampoo or conditioner when you purchase a 32-ounce shampoo or conditioner.*

Sandy: *I would like to have another treatment, and that scalp massage sounds great, John. Do you have time to do it today?*

John: *Let me check my schedule . . . yes. Here is what we will do. I will cut your hair first, then Marc can do your treatment and scalp massage. I'll finish your hair afterward.*

Sandy: *Sounds great to me.*

Salon scripts can eliminate miscommunication, which is the primary reason that clients don't come back to a salon

Increasing Retail Sales

Scripting increases sales at the checkout. How many times has your client forgotten to get retail products because you didn't follow through at the reception desk? An exiting script for the client helps prevent stylists from forgetting to give the client the suggested retail products.

The stylist escorts the client to the retail center, where she gives the recommended products to the client. The stylist might say something like, "This is the shampoo and conditioner I recommended for you, and here is the styling glaze. For hairspray, we have two that would work well on your hair: one that is firm hold and the other a working spray. Which one do you prefer?"

Retaining Clients

Salon scripts can eliminate miscommunication, which is the primary reason that clients don't come back to a salon, and thus help a salon achieve higher client retention rates.

Client (Madaline): *I really dislike long nails.*

Nail tech Carolyn: (paraphrases to clarify what the client said): *Are you saying that you would like your nails a little shorter?*

Madaline: *Oh, no. My length is OK. I just don't like them as long as that last client you did.*

Imagine what would have happened if Carolyn hadn't paraphrased Madaline's comment. Carolyn might have assumed that Madaline wanted shorter nails and filed them down before Madaline could stop her. Carolyn could have lost her client.

Soothing Displeased Clients

Salon scripts help stylists retain even displeased clients. Perhaps you hope a client won't be back, but if that's not the case, a salon script can help you keep that client.

Client Louise:	*This color you did is all wrong for me. It makes my skin look sallow.*
Colorist Robert:	*Sounds like you're angry about your haircolor. I'm sorry to hear that.*
Louise:	*You bet I'm angry. I want it fixed right now. I want my color back to the red I always wear.*
Robert:	*What you're saying is that this color is different from your regular red. Is that true?*
Louise:	*Yes, my usual color isn't this orange.*
Robert:	*If I could fix it today, would you have the time?*

Salon dialogue is more than selling retail and services; it's saying the right words to a client at the right time, including when a client isn't happy.

The Exit Dialogue

Planning your client's future visits is a vital key to client retention

Scripting an exit dialogue ensures that the client leaves the salon looking forward to the next visit. Planning your client's future visits is a vital key to client retention.

Esthetician Suzanne: *The paraffin treatment I did today is the best way to moisturize your skin. However, during your skin analysis, I noticed your skin would benefit from deep-*

exfoliating AHA treatments. AHA treatments would remove the dead skin cell layers, which can act as a barrier to deep moisturizing.

Client Sheri: *I've heard of AHA, but I didn't understand how it worked.*

Suzanne: *AHA, or Alpha Hydroxy Acid makes your skin look younger by refining the texture. When the excess skin cells are exfoliated, wrinkles are softer looking. AHA reduces the appearance of fine lines.*

Sheri: *It really does sound like something I need. I'll have to try it sometime.*

Suzanne: *You can purchase one treatment at a time. However, the most beneficial way to have AHA treatments is to do a series of six treatments about a week apart. If you purchase the whole series, you will get a free facial.*

Sheri: *Free facial . . . that's a great deal!*

Suzanne: *I work Tuesday and Thursday evenings, so you can get the treatments after work if you would like. Would you like to start the series next week, or would the following week fit better into your schedule?*

When you discuss all the exciting changes you can do with your client's next color service, haircut, nails, or skin care, she will be more likely to schedule immediately for her next appointment.

Using Questions to Enhance Sales

Controlling Questions

The person asking the question is the person in control. A question takes control of your mind, with or without your permission. If I asked you "Which teams do you think will make it to

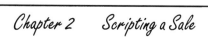

the Superbowl this year?" some of you would immediately think of two teams. Everyone else who didn't have an answer would start searching their mind for one—even if they weren't interested in football. The point is that everyone responds to the question involuntarily. A question, no matter what kind or content, takes control of the other person's mind. Asking the right questions put us in control of the client/stylist communication.

Leading Questions

The most effective way of starting conversations that command your client's attention is to ask a leading question containing a tempting offer. Your opening remark should cause the client to need to know about your product and should answer the client's question, "Why should I listen to you?" Here are some examples:

How would you like to have your nails look great for two weeks with practically no maintenance?

Would you be interested in a product that is guaranteed to give your hair more body?

Would you be interested in a new perm service that gives your hair curl that looks like natural wave without damage to your hair?

Wouldn't you love to have skin that feels like it did when you were a child?

Using a leading question "enrolls" your client in decision making and makes it much easier for you to focus on your client's needs and close the sale.

Open and Closed Questions

There are two types of questions that get different kinds of results. To get as much information as possible from clients, ask open questions. To get short, yes or no answers, use closed questions.

Open: *How do you care for your hair?*

Closed: *Do you style your hair everyday?*

Open: *Why do you think your hair is breaking?*

Closed: *Is your hair breaking because of this perm?*

Open: *What problems have you had when you style your own hair?*

Closed: *Do you have trouble styling your hair at home?*

Open: *What improvement would you like to see in you hair?*

Open: *What kind of perms have you had during the past two years?*

Closed: *Have you had any perms during the past two years?*

Using Questions to Take Control

When you want to command the attention of someone and be sure their mind wanders as little as possible, tag a question at the end of every three to five statements. Here are some sample tag questions:

> Your hair is really straight, isn't it?
>
> Are you with me?
>
> Does that make sense?
>
> You want your style to be as easy as possible, isn't that right?

Anytime you feel like you are losing control of the conversation, ask a question.

You can enhance sales by asking different types of questions. Asking the right questions put us in control of the client/stylist communication.

Yes Questions

When you are serious about selling, ask a series of questions that require a yes answer. Creating the client yes mode carries through to the closing of the sale. Here are some sample yes questions:

> Those few streaks of blonde around your face do brighten your complexion, don't they?
>
> Do you see how much fullness you have on top?

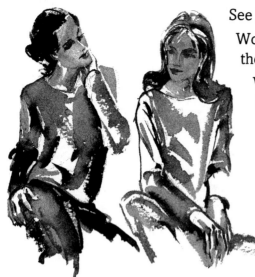

See how I use this thermal brush to smooth out the curl?

Wouldn't you agree that your hair looks thicker now that the ends are trimmed?

Would you like to have more body and shine in your hair?

Does your hair go flat easily?

Isn't it amazing that we can make fine hair have this much volume?

Can you see how many ways you can use this styling glaze?

Would you like your style to hold better?

Would you like your style to be versatile?

If you can get a series of six yes answers, you can get the sale.

Closing the Sale

Without sales we would all be out of business. How often do you inform your client of all the benefits of owning a product and then fail to close the sale at the last moment? Because no one likes to be turned down, it's human nature to avoid asking for the sale. If you are uncomfortable asking for a sale, there are many popular closes that guide a client to yes, some that let you avoid the direct asking part of closing a sale. Some examples are as follows:

Direct request: *Can we go ahead and do your manicure today?*

Assume the client is going to buy: *I'm going to go ahead and put the (product) on the front desk for you. Or, I'm going to go ahead and tell the receptionist to schedule you for that paraffin treatment next week.*

Forced choice: *Would Tuesday evening or Wednesday afternoon be the best time for your highlight? Or, This is the styling glaze I used to give your hair more body. Would you like to have the 8-ounce or the 16-ounce size?*

If I could, would you: *If I could find time today, would you like to have a décolleté treatment with your facial?*

No matter how great a salesperson you are, some clients will always have objections to sales. Sales resistance is often caused by a lack of information during the sales presentation. Objections can be overcome when the client has been shown enough benefits to purchase the product.

A common sales objection is that a product is too expensive.

Sales resistance is often caused by a lack of information during the sales presentation.

Stylist: *I know how you feel. You're absolutely right, ours does seem expensive. However, this shampoo and conditioner will save you money in the long run. With regular use, your hair will be in better condition and your color should last longer. You'll save time because your hair will be more manageable. Besides, this is very concentrated and will cost you only about 10 cents a day. That's pretty affordable, isn't it?*

Sometimes a client's objection is "I'll wait to buy the product."

Stylist/manager Diane: *Wouldn't you like to get this much body in your hair at home?*

Annette: *Yes, but I just bought a 16-ounce Marvella setting gel at the beauty supply store. I'll wait until I finish that and then buy your gel.*

Diane: *The gel you have is probably a high-quality gel; however, it may not have the features you need for your fine hair. Didn't you say that you have trouble with your hair going flat?*

Annette: *Yes, I suppose that could be because of the gel.*

Diane: *If you're not satisfied with this styling glaze, bring it back. We have an unconditional guarantee.*

Sometimes a client's objection is "I'll think it over."

Stylist John: *You wouldn't think it over if you weren't really interested. Maybe you're unsure because I didn't explain the process thoroughly. To clarify my thinking, are you concerned about damaging your hair with the perm?*

Client Patty: *Well yes, that's part of it. I'm also worried that I'll get too much curl. You know, like I had when I got the last perm.*

To overcome objections, first identify them. Then ask open questions to find out the underlying reasons the client resists purchasing. Perhaps you didn't explain the product or service thoroughly or present the benefits persuasively enough. Remember, never pressure, always persuade.

Professional Sales vs. High-Pressure Sales

Most salon professionals object to being called salespeople primarily because they don't like high-pressure sales. When they think of high-pressure sales they think of the insistent salesperson in the carpet store, the insurance salesperson, or the salesperson who goes door to door selling vacuum cleaners. In most cases, high-pressure salespeople aren't looking past the next paycheck. Since the slogans "a sale at any cost" and "buyer beware" characterize the personality of high-pressure salespeople, it is no wonder that salon professionals cringe at the word *sales*.

Good salespeople are persistent, not pushy, and know the difference between the two, which can turn a one-time sale into a long-term client. There are five main differences between high-pressure sales and professional sales.

1. High-pressure salespeople talk most of the time. Professional salespeople are just the opposite. They listen most of the time and talk primarily to answer the client's questions or to ask open-ended questions that keep the client talking. Professionals concentrate on what the client is saying rather than thinking about what to say next. Professionals are interested in what the client needs, and you can't find that out unless you stop talking and begin listening.

Jennifer just finished cutting Jason's hair and is suggesting that he purchase some retail products. Jason is a college student who gets a haircut every two months. At the reception desk, Jennifer places the recommended products on the counter.

Jennifer: *Jason, this is the shampoo and treatment that will tame that curly hair of yours. And this is the finishing creme. This shampoo is specially formulated to put moisture back in naturally dry hair like yours. It has sea kelp in it and amodimethicone and amino acids. I know you will love the way it works on your hair. It will make your hair more manageable and less susceptible to humidity changes. Wouldn't that be wonderful?*

Jason: *Yes, that would be great. How much does it cost?*

Jennifer: *Oh, Margo will tell you when she rings it up. I just know you will think it works miracles on your hair. It will save you a lot of time, too. You won't have to fight with your hair in the mornings. Just comb in the finishing creme and go.*

Jason: *I don't think I can afford all this stuff, Jennifer.*

Jennifer: *Oh, sure you can. I know you'll love it. Gotta go now. My next client is here. See you next month.*

Jason decided to wait until next time to buy the products. If Jennifer had listened and addressed the real objection, it is possible she could have saved the sale.

2. High-pressure salespeople push to conclude a sale while professionals work toward building a long-term relationship with the client. Retaining clients is the key to your future success. When your only interest is sales today at any cost, the client can tell. Clients learn quickly when you are concerned about their needs and when you are selling for the sake of sales. When you truly have your client's interest at heart, you will have a long-term selling relationship with that client.

3. Professionals are persistent, not insistent. When professionals know that a product or service is perfect for the client, they don't quit when the client rejects the sale. Neither are

Carol Lyden Smith

CLS Academy

Knoxville, TN

Carol is the president of CLS Academy in Knoxville, Tennessee, and is one of our industry's leading motivational speakers in sales and personal development. Her theory is that if you sell a product, you will have objections. If you sell a concept, there is no argument. Carol believes that the best way to sell to a client is to let them experience the benefits of that product. When the experience is beautiful and satisfying, the client can't resist.

they insistent that the client make the purchase. Real professionals let their clients know they have what the client needs and are prepared to serve them when the time comes.

Jennifer's client Mary is getting a new style. When the cut is finished, Jennifer begins to dry Mary's hair.

Shirley Shute

Educator

OPI

I truly believe that by educating the client on both products and services, she will have a better understanding of how professional salons can provide her with the excellence and quality she deserves. With an awareness how and why products work, clients will realize how important it is for them to purchase professional retail products to use at home.

Jennifer: *Your new cut would be much easier if you had a body wave in it. We could wave just the inside layers and let the outside fringe straight along your forehead, sides, and nape line. If I have time in my schedule today, would you like to go ahead and get the body wave? If you get a perm and cut together, it costs a little less than doing it separately. It's called a multiservice discount.*

Mary: *Oh, I don't know Jennifer, I haven't had a perm in years. I'd really rather see how the cut works without a perm first.*

Jennifer: *Wouldn't it be nice to dry your hair and not have to fight with it?*

Mary: *I know I always complain about my straight hair, but I don't think I'm ready for a perm yet.*

Jennifer: *We can do perms now that will leave your hair soft and in beautiful condition. So if you are concerned about the condition, don't be. It will feel healthy.*

Mary: *Yes, I am concerned about damaged hair. But I'm more concerned about the curl. I had a perm a few years ago that was so curly I couldn't get it to stay down.*

Jennifer: *Oh, I'm sorry that happened to you. A perm doesn't have to be like that. We can perm it in very large rods so it has just a gentle wave.*

Mary: *Let me think about it.*

Jennifer: *Remember, Mary, that when you wore the longer style you could pull your hair up if it wasn't working the way you wanted it to. But now, with short hair, it could be really frustrating in the morning to get it styled the way you want it. Seriously, think about a perm. Your hair has great texture and I know it would perm just like natural curl.*

Mary: *Maybe it would—but I'm just not ready yet.*

Jennifer:	OK. I'll show you how to use the curling iron to style your new cut. If you want to get permed within the next two weeks, I'll still give you the discount.
Mary:	How much discount do I get?
Jennifer:	It's about 10 percent, I think. Do you want me to find out exactly?
Mary:	No, I'll check with Margo at the desk when I leave. You said two weeks?
Jennifer:	Yes, two weeks.
Mary:	Maybe I'll schedule a body wave for next week. By then I'll know if I really need it or not and we can go from there.
Jennifer:	That sounds good, Mary. I'm sure you'll love having a perm.

4. High-pressure salespeople sell based on what they presume a client needs instead of the client's real needs. Clients don't care that your product will make hair curlier if their concern is that they are becoming bald. Your goal as a professional is to find out the client's needs and to place your product within those needs.

Suzanne, the salon's esthetician, rushes to the reception desk.

Suzanne:	Margo, did that last client of mine buy those two new masks I recommended?
Margo:	No, she didn't, Suzanne. She said she didn't have time to do all that to her face. She wants something a little simpler.
Suzanne:	Well why didn't she tell me? I could have recommended something else.
Margo:	Well, maybe you should have listened to her a little more. It was obvious to me when she was at the desk that she is a very busy professional woman and doesn't have an hour a week to mask her face.
Suzanne:	You don't have to beat me up, Margo. I guess I'm so excited about this new product I think everyone should use it. She did tell me she didn't have time for extended skin

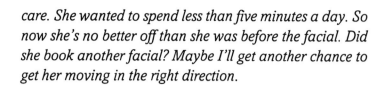

care. She wanted to spend less than five minutes a day. So now she's no better off than she was before the facial. Did she book another facial? Maybe I'll get another chance to get her moving in the right direction.

Suzanne's push to sell products that obviously don't fit into the customer's lifestyle could alienate the client enough that she doesn't return. At best, the client will come back but will be cautious about Suzanne's future recommendations.

5. Professionals show clients real value while high-pressure salespeople push specials and discounts. Long-term customers are more interested in value and quality than price. Specials and discounts are incentives to induce additional sales when you already have a relationship with a client. When customers buy because of price, it is likely that they will only buy when there is a discount or special, and they will switch to your competition as soon as they find a better deal.

To lure new customers into their business, unknowing hair salons will run an ad in the newspaper for a permanent wave at a discount. Usually, the only customers they attract are their current clients or the people who take advantage of the discount but don't return until the next time a perm is offered at a discount. It is true that some salons exist by offering discounts. However, to build long-term clients, sell value and quality, and then offer specials as an added incentive.

Chapter Summary

1. What you say and how you say it have significant impact on your professional growth. Voice tone, body language, and choosing the best words are some of the basic skills you must master to become a captivating communicator.

2. Salon scripts help establish trust between the client and the stylist.

3. Scripting increases the awareness of available salon services.

4. Scripting increases sales at the checkout.

5. Scripting increases client retention rates.

6. Scripting dialogue helps stylists to retain even displeased clients.

7. Scripting an exit dialogue ensures that the client leaves the salon looking forward to her next visit.

8. Open questions are used to get a client to talk more. Closed questions are used when you want a simple yes or no answer.

9. The best salespeople ask a series of questions that require a yes answer from the client. Creating the client yes mode carries through to the closing of the sale.

10. Closing the sale is the most important part of the sales process. Because no one likes to be turned down, it's common to avoid the final request for the sale. There are easy scripts that can help you breeze your way through closing a sale.

11. Sales resistance is often caused by a lack of information during the sales presentation. Objections can be overcome when the client has been shown enough benefits to purchase the product.

12. Good salespeople are persistent, not pushy, and know the difference between the two, which can turn a one-time sale into a long-term client.

13. One difference between high-pressure salespeople and professionals is that high-pressure salespeople push to conclude a sale while professionals work toward building a long-term relationship with the client.

14. Professional salespeople are persistent, not insistent. When professionals know that a product or service is perfect for the client, they don't quit when the client rejects the sale.

15. Professionals show clients real value while high-pressure salespeople push specials and discounts. Long-term customers are more interested in value and quality than price.

16. Professional salespeople listen most of the time and talk primarily to answer the client's questions or to ask open-ended questions that keep the client talking. Professionals concentrate on what the client is saying rather than thinking about what to say next.

Creating a Script

Features and Benefits of Products

Consumers are motivated to buy for two basic reasons: to feel good and to solve problems. If you buy a light bulb, chances are you are buying it to solve a problem—you need light. When you purchase the light bulb, you have many choices with many features. You can choose a light bulb that uses less energy, one that has soft light, or one that has three different wattages. A product's features create a picture in the consumer's mind. However, the real motivation to buy is in the benefits. You buy the light bulb because of what it will do for you. It will save you money, give you the choice of subdued light for relaxing or bright light for reading, and it is easy on your eyes. You make a purchase because of the benefits rather than the features. The benefits answer the question, "What will this purchase do for me?" Perhaps you think you buy a new outfit because of the features (the color, the design, the quality of fabric), but would you make that purchase if you didn't feel good wearing the outfit? Features account for about 20% of your decision to purchase, and benefits are responsible for the remaining 80%.

To differentiate between features and benefits, remember that features are the product's characteristics, such as the size, ingredients, and purpose. If you were buying a car, some of its features would be cruise control, CD player, a sun roof, and leather seats. When you think about those features, your mind is directed to the feelings created by those features. When you think about cruise control, you feel how great it would be to take your foot off the accelerator and let the car drive itself. When a CD player is mentioned, you see yourself driving along listening to your favorite music. Leather seats invoke a feeling of sinking into soft and pliable leather. When a sun roof is mentioned, you find yourself thinking about a summer day and the breeze coming in through the open sun roof. You hear or see features, and you feel the benefits.

The features of a wheat strengthening shampoo would be as follows:

It is available in 4-, 8-, 16-, or 32-ounce sizes.

It is concentrated.

It contains hydrolyzed keratin and hydrolyzed wheat protein.

It contains natural nutrients and restores natural shine.

It cleanses thoroughly and eliminates limpness.

The benefits are what the client gains from purchasing the product. They answer the question, "Does the product make the client feel good or solve the client's problems?" Since the benefits of a product or service are derived from its features, you must first know the features in order to offer the benefits to your customer. Remember, sales motivation is in the benefits.

Learn to talk to customers in terms of benefits. Use the following words to describe benefits to your client:

Features of a product account for about 20% of a customer's decision to purchase, and benefits are responsible for the remaining 80%.

adds manageability

controls

fashionable

beauty

sex appeal

healthy hair

nourishes

gives body and fullness

saves money

saves time

strengthens

adds shine

eliminate frizzies

softens

look younger

easier

feels great

lasts longer

revitalized

luxurious

won't damage

attractive

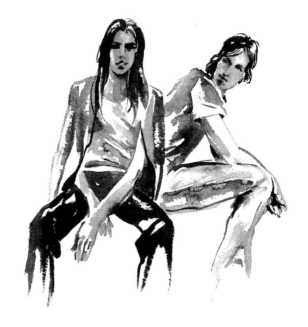

Now look again at the features for wheat strengthening shampoo and match the benefits to the features.

Features of Wheat Strengthening Shampoo	Benefits
Comes in 4-, 8-, 16-, or 32-ounce sizes	Convenient sizes
Concentrated	Lasts longer
Contains hydrolyzed keratin and hydrolyzed wheat protein	Strong, shiny hair
Strengthens hair	Adds body
	Thicker-looking hair
Cleanses thoroughly	Gives hair volume
Contains natural ingredients	Healthy
Eliminates limpness	Easy to style
	Saves time
	Attractive hair
	Restores natural shine

A product's features are easy to find. Manufacturers list them in their product literature and on their labels.

Without looking at the bottle or any literature about the product, think of your favorite salon product, preferably one that you have been using for a few years. List five features of that product. Remember that features are the product's characteristics. Then list the benefits of those features.

Features	Benefits
1	
2	
3	
4	
5	

Did you discover that remembering the features was more difficult than remembering the benefits? If this is your favorite product, you use it because of its benefits, not because of its features. Once you figured out the features, the benefits were easy. Write down the features and benefits of every product you use in your salon. Knowing and understanding your products will help you sell services as well as products.

Stylist Monique: *While I'm styling your hair today, I will show you a few easy tips to help you do your hair at home. These tips will give you the manageability and fullness that I think you are looking for. I think they will also cut down on the time you have to spend on your hair each day.*

Client: *That sounds too good to be true, Monique. Show me what you've got.*

Monique: *I will be using these three products: wheat protein for volume, styling glaze to give your hair body, and finishing spray to hold the style. I'll also show you how much of each to use.*

Client: *OK, go on.*

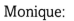

Monique: *First, apply the wheat protein. Work it in. In fact, it's a good idea to massage it into your scalp. Feel how it stimulates?*

Client: *Yes. It feels cool.*

Monique: *Now use about four pumps of styling glaze. One on the back of your head, each side, and on top. Work it through your hair. Now*

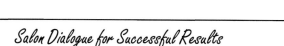

watch how I use the brush to dry and create volume at the same time.

Monique   (after explaining entire styling procedure):   *See how much volume you can get by using the wheat protein and styling glaze? It really looks great.*

Client: *Will this hold up through tonight? It's awfully damp outside.*

Monique: *Watch how I use the finishing spray. If you lift the hair and spray underneath, the finishing spray will support your style better.*

Client: *It does look great. Thanks for all the styling tips.*

Monique: *You're welcome. I'm glad you like it. I'll show you where those products are in the reception area.*

Features and Benefits of Services

In the past, in product knowledge classes it has been commonplace to learn the features and benefits of products. Today, with the variety of services to offer clients, it is as important to learn the features and benefits of services. If you object to "selling to your client," think of it as giving clients the information they need to make an informed decision. Writing out the features and benefits of services is the prelude to writing a salon script.

If you object to "selling to your client," think of it as giving clients the information they need to make an informed decision.

Creating a Script

Scripts can be used in every area of your business. They can be used to sell a particular product, such as a skin care product, or a concept, such as a gift certificate for a spa package; as a tool to train new salon professionals; or for salon special promotions. Scripts can also be used to create a consistency throughout a

Dry Skin Facial Treatment

Features	Benefits
Two cleansings with cleanser for your skin type	Deep cleanses skin
Use of a papaya enzyme mask to remove dead skin cells	Smoother skin
Includes a facial massage	
Relieves stress	Relaxes and relieves stress
A three-layer paraffin mask	Deep moisturizes skin

Permanent Wave

Features	Benefits
Curls hair	Hair looks more attractive
Lasts for months	Great value
	Saves money
Odorless	Pleasant experience
Holds set from shampoo to shampoo	Saves time
Soft, natural-looking curl	Beautiful hair, hair feels great

Leg Waxing

Features	Benefits
Removes superfluous hair	Don't have to shave or tweeze
Hair grows back slowly	Saves time and energy
Hair grows back soft	Feels good, no stubble
Safe and easy on skin	No irritation/feels good

Sculptured Nails

Features	Benefits
Durable, tough	Strong and long-lasting
Polish stays on for two weeks	Saves time
Nails always the same length	Always look good
Can have long nails no matter how fragile your natural nails	Attractive hands
Smoothes out rough, uneven nails	Perfect nails

salon so that everyone says the same thing. All scripts have a common thread—they are all geared to selling to a client. You are either selling a product or service, your skills, or your salon.

Salon scripts become a permanent part of your salon policies and procedures. They sell and reinforce your salon image to your client. An example of a salon script is your receptionist's telephone greeting to clients and your stylists' methods of introducing new clients to the salon.

Salon Script for New Clients

Marc: *Good morning, Heidi. My name is Marc and I will be your stylist today.*

Heidi: *Hello, Marc, it's nice to meet you.*

Marc: *Before we get started, I want to take just a minute to show you around our salon and explain the salon brochure to you.*

Heidi: *That sounds good. I'd like to see the salon.*

Marc: *Our salon has been here for eighteen years, and just two years ago we expanded into a day spa. As you can see in your brochure, we offer full service hair, nail, and skin care and many different types of body services. On the next page of your brochure you have a description of all the spa packages we offer.*

Heidi: *Wow. I didn't know you did all this!*

Marc: *Yes, and in addition to the spa packages, we also have bridal packages. That's on the next page. If you'll follow me, I'll take you on a quick tour and then we will sit down and talk about your hair.*

While on the tour, Marc mentions all the features of the salon services and the benefits that Heidi could have by taking advantage of those services.

All salon scripts should have a common thread—they are all geared to selling to a client. You are either selling a product or service, your skills, or your salon.

Service Scripts

Once you have established a script for the various services, they will change slowly, only as techniques change and improve.

Scripts for services can remain unchanged for long periods of time. Once you have established a script for the various services, they will change slowly, only as techniques change and improve.

Marc: *Heidi, you say that you would like to have a your hair cut as short as the haircut in this picture?*

Heidi: *Yes, I had it that short before and I really liked it, except that I had to shampoo it too often. I'd rather not have to style it every day.*

Marc: *If I could create the look you want so that you don't have to style it every day, would you like that?*

Heidi: *Why yes, I would. How could you do that?*

Marc: *We could give you a body perm. I guarantee that it will look just like natural curl. It will be soft and shiny. The wave will give you the support you need just where you need it. Wouldn't you like to have a little extra body in your hair?*

Heidi: *Yes. I'd love to have more body in my hair, but I am afraid a perm will be frizzy.*

Marc: *Perms today are very gentle and I would use large perm rods so that the curl pattern is big and soft. You have great hair, so I imagine a perm in your hair would last about four months.*

Heidi: *How much does it cost?*

Marc: *You only need rods in the top and crown, so we wouldn't be doing a full perm. The cost would be around $40.00 in addition to your haircut. That would work out to be about $2.50 a week. Not bad for something that saves you thirty minutes two or three times a week.*

Heidi: *You're right. If it saves me that much time, it's surely worth it. Do you have time to do it today?*

Product Scripts

Product scripts are usually considered permanent. New scripts must be written when the product is improved or when new products are introduced. Create your own folder of product features and benefits by collecting all the written material from manufacturers about their products. Then write at least five benefits for each product. Your retail sales will increase dramatically if you can give your client at least five reasons why he or she should buy the product.

Marc: *Heidi, I want to show you how to style your new haircut and perm. First, I'll use this styling gel. It's strong enough to hold your set for a few days. It helps shine and condition hair naturally. You can see by the ingredients that it contains many natural plant extracts. Use about this much* (Marc puts gel into the palm of his hand and then applies it to Heidi's hair). *Watch how I use my fingers to lift the hair in your crown. Just lift the hair and move it back toward the center.*

    Now that your hair is dry, I'll use some finishing creme to control and smooth the sides and nape area. Just put a small amount into your palms, like this. Rub your palms together and then smooth your hair with your hands. The finishing creme is a light hold, and it protects your hair from dryness. See how shiny and soft your hair is. The perm works beautifully, you just won't believe how easy it will be to style your hair. Doesn't it seem to have a lot of body?

Heidi: *It looks great, Marc. I'm so glad you had time to do the perm.*

Marc: *Excellent. Glad you like it. I'll get your gel and finishing creme for you at the reception desk while you go change into your clothes.*

Margo: *Hello, Heidi. I love your new style. Marc does a great job, doesn't he?*

Heidi: *Yes. I love it, too. Marc, did you get that gel for me?*

Marc: *I have the gel right here and the finishing creme. I know you already have professional shampoo and conditioner at home, but I want you to change conditioners now. With your perm, you should use a more moisturizing conditioner, at least until the end of winter. Here, this one will be the best.*

Heidi: *OK, I'll try it, but get me the small one please till I see if I like it.*

Promotional Scripts

Promotional scripts change with each salon promotion, which in many salons is every six weeks. These promotions are the most challenging and most rewarding. They can be stimulating to those salon professionals who like to compete in sales contests or against their own past performance. In the following dialogue, Margo, the receptionist, is working on a promotion designed to build clientele for the estheticians and sell products for the skin care department.

Promotional scripts change with each salon promotion, which in many salons is every six weeks.

Margo: *Heidi, we are having a special promotion for this month. Since you have purchased more than twenty-five dollars in products, you may have a free skin analysis by one of our estheticians. When would you like to schedule for that? It will take approximately twenty minutes.*

Heidi: *Free skin analysis? I don't have to buy anything?*

Margo: *No, you don't have to buy anything. The esthetician will cleanse your skin and examine it. Then she will tell you what treatments and products would best benefit your skin.*

Heidi: *I have never had a skin analysis. It sounds like fun. Can I get a time early next week?*

Parts of a Script

A script has seven main parts:

Purpose: Goal of the script

Opening: Greeting; building rapport

Proposal: Specifically what are you selling?

Features: What are the features of the offer?

Benefits: What does the client get out of it?

Close: Ask for the sale.

Exit: Prepare for future sales; thank the client.

A script flowchart helps simplify a script and makes it easy to use. At a glance, salon staff can read and learn the different parts of a script using a flowchart. A flowchart should be used for all scripts.

Purpose

Specifically write out the goal of your script. The goal could be to increase the sale of skin care products by 500 units per month during the next three months. The goal could be to create a script to introduce clients to the salon, or a script that creates a consistent way of answering the phone or scheduling appointments.

Opening

Creating a great first impression is imperative in attaining sales. Take time to greet your clients and build rapport before beginning your sales script. Be sure clients are comfortable. Respect your clients' time, and be certain your atmosphere is conducive to good listening. Building rapport means finding common interests that allow you to get to know your clients. Don't rush into the sale. Get clients talking first so you can find out what they need. If you are making an offer on the phone, be careful about taking up too much of your clients' time. Keep it short and sweet.

Proposal

Specifically what is the offer? If it is a service or sales promotion, keep it simple and familiar: for example, "buy one, get one half price," "free gift with purchase," or perhaps a simple introductory offer. (If the proposal is "buy one skin care product and get the second half price," of course the lowest priced item is half price.) The offer could be time limited: for example, "offer expires on March 31." Or it could be more specific: for example, "Cold weather barrier serum will be half price when purchased with your choice of moisturizers."

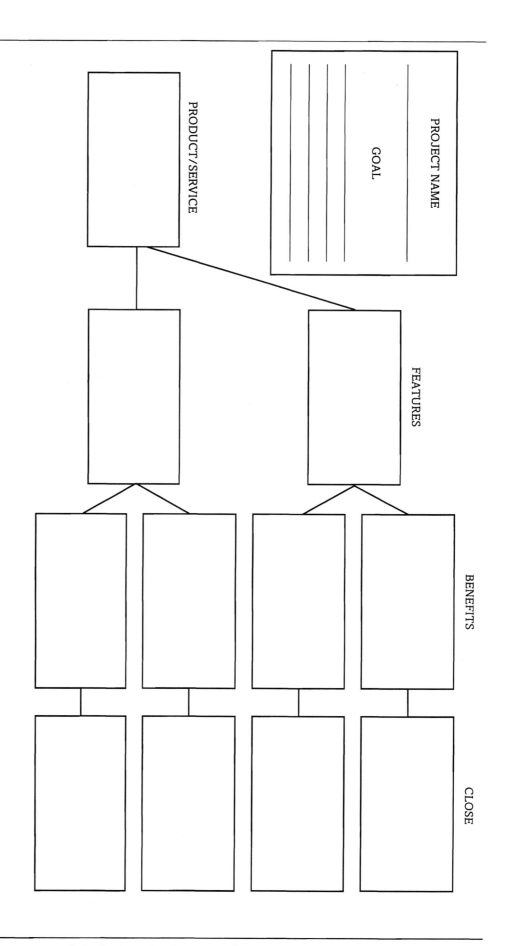

PROJECT NAME

GOAL

PRODUCT/SERVICE

FEATURES

BENEFITS

CLOSE

Features

Using manufacturers' information in addition to knowledge gained by your experience with the product, write down all the product's features. If you are selling a service, you will create the features from your experience.

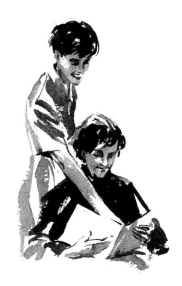

Benefits

After the features are listed, the benefits are easy. The more benefits you offer, the easier it is to sell the product or service.

Closing

List all the closes you can use for your script. Since no two people are stimulated to buy in the same way, you need many different closes to choose from. Using the right closing technique can mean the difference between getting and closing the sale. If you don't ask for the order, there is no sale.

The Exit

The exit is a wrap-up, a summary that also gives salon professionals a chance to plan future sales and/or services for clients. It is also a reminder to give a genuine thank you to the client for purchasing and a warm good-bye.

Composing a Script Book

One way to bring scripting into daily use is to create a script book that arms you with answers to your clients' strongest objections. It's important to answer all questions and concerns accurately and intelligently. The more information you have at your fingertips, the less likely you will be at a loss for words.

The first step is to identify common objections, such as the following:

PRODUCT/SERVICE

Introductory offer:
New Body Building Styling Lotion
Purchase 32 ounces at regular cost,
$16.95, and get 4-ounces hairspray at
half price.

PROJECT NAME
Body Building Styling Lotion
Special Offer
Goal: Sell 30 each week for
4 weeks, 120 total

FEATURES

Concentrated
Great value
Recyclable containers
No product buildup

Contains wheat and corn
proteins
Contains panthenol
Contains algae extract
No alcohol

BENEFITS

Save money
Convenient, lasts a long time
Environmentally friendly
Won't weigh hair down

Strengthens hair
Makes hair more pliable
Moisturizes and provides
humidity control

Makes hair shiny and adds
elasticity
Won't dry out your hair

Holds style better
Adds body to all hair types
Adds resilience to style

CLOSE

How many would you like?

I'll put the styling lotion on the
front desk for you. Do you have
enough shampoo and conditioner
till next time or should I get
some for you today?

This is the lotion I used on you
today.
See how much body you have
now?

- I want to use up what I have first.
- What can I get at the drug store?
- It's too expensive.
- I don't have enough time.
- I want to think about it.
- I don't need it right now.
- I like what I'm using now.
- I'll get it next time.
- Someday I'll indulge myself.

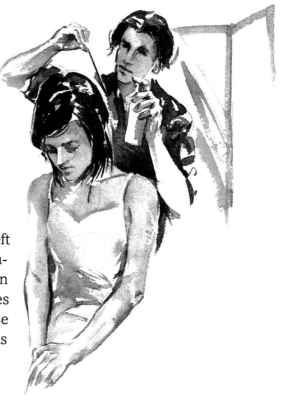

Use two pages for each objection. On the left side, use the objection as a header. Then list the answers under the objection. An average salesperson would list three to five answers; however, top sales performers list ten to fifteen responses. Finally, use the opposite page of your script book for comments from actual experiences of the objection.

Script Book Example

Objection	Actual Experiences
"I want to use up what I have at home first"	Recommending a conditioner for Mrs. Ramsay.
• How long will it last? Are you sure it will last until your next service?	Facial moisturizers for Janice Stringer
• The products I recommend will improve the manageability of your hair. Wouldn't you like to see those improvements right away?	
• Can you see that your hair has more body now with this styling lotion?	
• Wouldn't you like to have shinier hair now?	
• Wouldn't you like to have smoother skin now?	
• Isn't there anyone else in your family who could use the products you already have at home?	

Here are some more objections and answers.

Objection: *I want to use up what I have first.*

Answers: *How long will it last? Are you sure it will last until your next service?*

The products I recommend will improve the manage-ability of your hair. Wouldn't you like to see those improvements right away?

Can you see that your hair has more body now with this styling lotion?

Wouldn't you like to have shinier hair now?

Wouldn't you like to have smoother skin now?

Isn't there anyone else in your family who could use the products you already have at home?

I must not have explained the product properly to you. I know if I had you wouldn't leave here without this product. What questions do you still have?

Objection: *What can I get at the drug store?*

Answers: *There are probably some satisfactory products that you can purchase at a discount or drug store. However, the products I recommend for you are formulated for your hair (skin, nail) type. You will get the best results from them.*

Are you concerned about price? (Refer to answers for the "It's too expensive" objection.)

Is it more convenient for you to go to a drug store?

Objection: *It's too expensive.*

Answers: *As compared to what?*

Did I explain how concentrated this product is?

Did you know that this product costs just pennies a day to use?

Long-term use of this product will save you money. Because your hair will have more body, you will be able to use less styling lotion. Doesn't that make sense?

This nail polish may cost more, but it will last much longer than other brands, and it strengthens your nails at the same time.

It may cost more than other products, but there is no comparison in quality.

You can use your credit card if that will make it easier.

Objection: *I don't have enough time.*

Answers: *When would you have time?*

May I tell you the ways that other clients like you create the time they need?

If I showed you how to save time with this product (service), would you do it?

Objection: *I want to think about it.*

Answers: *Do you mind telling me what it is you have to think about?*

Great. Let's think out loud. What are your concerns?

OK. What additional information do you need?

All right, what prevents you from buying?

I'm sorry. I must not have explained the product (service) thoroughly. What do you need to think about?

Objection: *I don't need it right now.*

Answers: *I must not have explained the product (service) thoroughly. If I had, you would see the value in buying today. Let me review it for you.*

Do you see how the quality of your skin has improved by using this moisturizer just one time? When do you think you will need it?

Wouldn't you like to have your skin look this good all the time?

Wouldn't you like to have stronger nails right away?

Wouldn't you like to start enjoying the benefits right away?

Objection: *I like what I'm using now.*

Answers: *If I remember correctly, you said you wanted your hair to have more shine. Is that correct? This is the product to do that for you.*

We talked about how dry your hands were, remem-

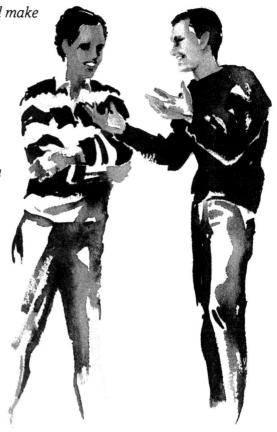

ber? It has been my experience that this lotion helps dryness better than any other lotion.

I have many clients with the same hair type. This is what they find to be the most effective product.

Does your product give you this much body and manageability?

Objection: *I'll get it next time.*

Answers: *Wouldn't you like to start enjoying the benefits right away?*

Why wait?

Specifically, what objections do you have?

Can you see the improvement in the texture of your hair? Wouldn't you like to reproduce that at home?

Objection: *Someday I'll indulge myself.*

Answers: *Purchasing professional conditioner isn't indulging yourself, Mrs. White, it is helpful and important to the health and appearance of your hair.*

Don't think of a facial as being self-indulgent. Think of it the same way you think about going to a dentist for a checkup and cleaning. Its purpose is preventative. The esthetician will deep clean your skin and teach you how to care for it better.

A scalp massage may seem a little indulgent, Mrs. White, however, your scalp needs some attention. I think you could stimulate hair growth with scalp massage.

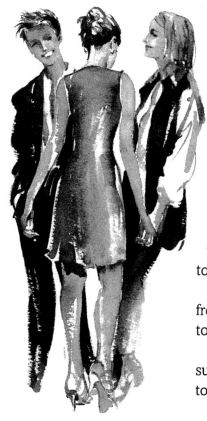

It doesn't take much experience as a salon professional to learn all the common objections people give for not buying a service or a product. Remember that clients often conceal their true concerns about your product. Only by listening carefully to your client's questions and comments will you find out the true basis of the objection. Then use open-ended questions to find out more about the objection.

If you have difficulty answering some objections, solicit help from your peers, managers, and even manufacturers' educators to find out how they have handled similar situations.

Scripts may make your presentation sound canned, so be sure to learn yours until they become natural. When you are able to answer your clients' objections and calm their fears of buying, you are just a close away from the sale. To make the greatest impact on future sales, use and update your script book regularly. A script book takes the stress and uncertainty out of selling. It will establish you as a competent professional and can put you miles ahead of your competition.

If you're not sold on your product or service yourself, sales will be impossible—unless, of course, your product sells itself. Similarly, you must be convinced that the product or service you are selling is of value to the client, or your client will hear the doubt in your voice. If you are in such a position, either find another product that you do like, or learn more about the one you are selling so that you can sell with integrity.

When you are able to answer your clients' objections and calm their fears of buying, you are just a close away from the sale.

Chapter Summary

1. Consumers are motivated to buy for two basic reasons: to feel good and to solve problems.

2. A product's features create a picture in the consumer's mind, but the real motivation to buy is the benefits.

3. Features are the product's characteristics, such as size, ingredients, and purpose. Benefits are what the client gains from purchasing the product, such as that it saves time, adds shine, or makes the skin or hair look healthier.

4. Today, with the variety of services to offer clients, it is as important to learn features and benefits of services as it is for products.

5. The main parts to a script are the purpose, which is the goal of the script, the opening, the proposal, the features, the benefits, the close, and the exit (the part of the script that prepares the client for future sales).

6. Salon scripts become a permanent part of your salon policies and procedures. They sell and reinforce your salon image to your client. An example of a salon script is your receptionist's telephone greeting to clients and your stylists' method of introducing new clients to the salon.

7. Your retail sales will increase dramatically if you can give your client at least five reasons why he or she should buy the product (or service).

8. Compose a script book of common objections and their answers so that you will never be at a loss for words.

9. The most common objections are, "I want to use up what I have first," "What can I get at the drug store?", "It's too expensive," "I don't have enough time," "I want to think about it," "I don't need it right now," "I like what I'm using now," and "I'll get it next time."

10. Remember that clients often conceal their true concerns about your product. Only by listening carefully to your client's questions and comments will you find out the true basis of the objection. Then use open-ended questions to find out more about the objection.

Chapter 4

Communication and People Types

*E*ach of us makes judgments about others. When you meet someone who looks, talks, and thinks the way you feel a person should, your body language and words will automatically indicate your approval of the other person. If, on the other hand, the person you meet is the antithesis of your ideal person, your reactions will indicate how you feel. Most of us expect others to act, think, talk, and look similar to us. If they don't, our automatic response is, "If they are different, they must be wrong."

If an elderly lady looks like your grandmother, you might think she will also have the same personality. If casual attire and a relaxed look are part of your lifestyle, you might not trust a man wearing a conservative suit.

It's easy to understand why we react this way. As we grow to adulthood, our environment and the people around us (primarily our parents) give us our life rules. Our life rules are our prejudices, our how to's and our do's and don'ts. As adults we use our life rules to make choices. For example, a person who was poor as a child might make the decision never to waste money. Another person with the same background might decide to enjoy his money because he never had it as a child.

All of the life rules that are stored in our memories are called tapes. When we live our lives according to our tape, we feel good about ourselves. When we see others live up to our tapes, we feel secure around them. When they don't, we feel threatened.

Unconditional Positive Regard

To be successful in the salon industry, where you are constantly in contact with varieties of people and personalities, it is good to understand Carl Rogers's concept of "unconditional positive regard." Simply stated, it means "to accept the many differences in other people's personality, appearance, beliefs, intelligence and decision making processes without judgment." (From Dr. Lew Loconcy, the New Psycosmetologist Seminar in Reading, PA 6/9–6/11, 1985.) It does not mean you must agree with someone else's view; it simply means that you accept that they have a different set of life rules. To accept unconditional positive regard is to accept that people are different and think differently.

When Life Rules Conflict

Conflict arises when two people's life rules are different. How you respond to those differences is up to you. One of Carolyn's life rules is to clean up during the day as she works. Carl learned his cleanup life rule from his father, who liked to let cleanup accumulate until the end of the day.

Carolyn: *Carl, you have color bowls all over the sink. Why don't you clean it up? It's a mess.*

Carl: *I'll get to it.*

Carolyn: *Yeah, I know you. You'll wait till I can't stand it any longer and I clean it up. Clean it up now, Carl.*

Carl: *Just leave it alone. I'll clean it up before I go home.*

Carolyn: *Oh Carl, you are impossible.*

Life rules get passed along, generation to generation, and when they are challenged we feel insecure. Some life rules remain valid through adulthood, and others become archaic as we mature. A rule that was established by young people in the 1960s was, "don't trust anyone over thirty." However, today those same young people are in their forties. Other archaic rules are "children should be seen and not heard," "every man who wears long hair uses drugs," or "all men with shaved heads are militant."

People are more susceptible to anger and conflict when they hang onto archaic life rules without objectively studying their tapes in light of new information. We call such people "stuck in their ways."

When You Talk to Yourself

Anytime you observe a situation, a dialogue takes place in your head to make sense of the situation from your viewpoint. You use your life rules to judge the situation.

One of your clients, Mrs. Smith, is scheduled with another stylist. You see on the appointment book that you could have taken the appointment. Several dialogues could take place in your head.

> "I wonder what I did wrong that Mrs. Smith would switch to Marc?"

> "How could that receptionist screw up so badly? She knows that Mrs. Smith is my customer."

> "Mrs. Smith is scheduled with Marc. I should check with Margo to be sure Mrs. Smith isn't scheduled wrong."

> "Well. I lost another one. I always lose clients. I work hard to give them what they want and then they switch to someone else. I might as well give up."

The tone of your internal dialogue is a result of the kind of memory tapes that are created by your life rules. They can affect you positively or negatively. If, as a child, you were told repeatedly that you were sloppy, you might live your entire life feeling that no matter what you do, you look sloppy. Feelings of inade-

Carlos Valenzuela
Phoenix, AZ

Carlos' latest audiotape series is Getting Results through Perception Management. *Perception management is based on the theory that everyone has a different view of things. Once you understand your own perceptions and learn about the other sixteen perceptions, you can appreciate the contribution that other people's perceptions make to your world. Only when everyone accepts that others' perceptions are important can they build an all-star team in which teamwork is truly effective in an organization.*

quacy are magnified by an internal dialogue that says, "I'm not good enough," or "I'm too fat," "I'm not good looking enough," or "I'm really dumb." Sometimes tapes such as these play in your mind so loudly that it becomes difficult or impossible to overcome them.

You can consciously change those internal messages when you hear them by replacing them with dialogue such as "I'm usually much neater than this," "I usually make better decisions than that," and "That isn't typical behavior for me."

The Way I See It

In a situation between two people, there are at least three different interpretations: "the way I see it," "the way you see it," and "the way it is." Sometimes all three are in agreement; however, that isn't the usual situation.

In the example of the client switching to another stylist, Jennifer, the stylist, perceives that Margo, the receptionist, is incompetent: "How could that receptionist screw up so badly? She knows that Mrs. Smith is my customer."

Margo's perception of the situation is, of course, totally different. She sees that she is doing her best to satisfy clients by scheduling Mrs. Smith with Marc. Mrs. Smith requested Jennifer; however, Jennifer's available time slot was a little too late. Mrs. Smith said she could make the later appointment time with Jennifer but then she would have to bring her children. She decided to take the appointment with Marc this time.

One of Jennifer's rules, "my clients belong to me," is showing. Margo's rule, "do what is best for the client," prompted her to schedule Jennifer's client with Marc.

Another co-worker, Carl, might see the situation in a different way from either Margo or Jennifer. In Carl's eyes, Margo should have first talked to Jennifer to see if she could squeeze in Mrs. Smith before she scheduled the appointment with Marc. Carl also doesn't understand why Jennifer is so upset.

Who is right? That's difficult to say. Regardless, there is a lack of communication, and without effort on both parts, the division will remain.

In a salon, you work closely with clients and co-workers. Your personal space is invaded regularly, and your personalities often bump into each other. Because intimacy is the nature of the salon industry, it is imperative that salon professionals learn to communicate feelings as well as words and concepts.

It is socially acceptable to demonstrate positive emotions, such as joy, optimism, and excitement; however, our society frowns on expression of negative emotions. When unexpressed negative emotions are allowed to build up (commonly called "stuffing") they can become explosive. Surfacing as anger, withdrawal, depression, anxiety, and worry, stuffing emotions create unhealthy environments that make others fear that they will be the target of the explosion.

The easiest way to avoid stuffing negative emotions is by remembering unconditional positive regard. By accepting the differences in others' thinking, you can change your expectations of them.

You may also collect negative emotions each time someone lets you down. If you set very high or very specific expectations for others, you may be disappointed often. Another way of collecting negative emotions is by thinking that other people automatically know what you want. You probably also assume that you know what they are thinking, again setting yourself up to collect negative feelings.

> *Because intimacy is the nature of the salon industry, it is imperative that salon professionals learn to communicate feelings as well as words and concepts.*

Diane the salon manager (talking to herself):   *Am I the only person here who cares if this place runs right? Can't anyone see that we're short of color and need to place an order? To me it's obvious that when there is only one tube of color left, someone should tell me so we can order it.*

Margo: *What did you say, Diane? I didn't hear you.*

Diane: *Oh, nothing. It's just the same old thing, Margo* (hands her the order). *Please place this color order right away.*

Margo: *You sound a little angry, Diane.*

Diane: *Yes, I am. We ran out of color again. I just don't know what that girl does with her time. I feel like she does this to me on purpose, just to make me angry.*

Margo: *Maybe you should talk to Janet about it. Maybe she doesn't understand what she is supposed to do.*

Diane: *I guess I could talk to her, but it won't do any good. She doesn't care.*

You can prevent negative emotion buildup by assuming that behind every behavior is positive intention and that when you need help, you should ask for it.

You can prevent negative emotion buildup by assuming that behind every behavior is positive intention and that when you need help, you should ask for it. The same situation, handled more rationally, would appear like this:

Diane: *Janet, we are short on color again. I need you to be more attentive to the inventory. How about if I go over the routine with you again?*

Janet: *I'm sorry, Diane. You're right, we are really short on color. I'll get an order together right away. It seems that I look at it one day and it looks fine, but the next day it's all gone. There has to be a better way of doing this.*

Diane: *It seems that you don't have a handle on it. We'll go over it again tonight after my last client.*

People Types

Depending on the situation, each of us responds in different ways. Because we have more than one expression of our personality, it is impossible to place people into types. However, to help understand personality differences between clients and co-workers, we have outlined some typical personalities and how to work with them.

The Spontaneous Personality

The spontaneous personality is driven by action. She tends to be impulsive, happy go lucky, and cheerful. Because a spontaneous personality doesn't like to schedule in advance, she is more likely to call the day she wants an appointment. If you can't take her, she will find another salon that will. In the unlikely event that she does schedule a few days ahead, she will often decide at the last minute to cancel her appointment because "something came up."

Part of the charm of the spontaneous personality is her impulsive leap toward new ideas, like changing her mind in the middle of a cut or deciding she wants a perm instead of a color.

When selling to a spontaneous personality, keep your presentation short and simple. Spontaneous characters buy impulsively and because they are not likely to pay attention to directions, be sure the instructions for product use are easy to read and understand.

The spontaneous co-worker can be an excellent team player and values equality rather than authoritarian work environments. Since the spontaneous co-worker learns by doing, she loves to attend hands-on workshops rather than lecture classes or shows. The spontaneous employee needs room and opportunities and flexibility to grow as opposed to structure and constraint.

A client arrives at Sensations Salon.

Margo: *Hello. How can I help you?*

Katrina: *I'm Katrina Katz. John usually cuts my hair. Does he have any time within the next hour or so?*

Margo: *I don't see any time available, but wait just a minute while I talk to him about it.*

(Margo excuses herself and goes off to find John.)

Margo: *John, Katrina is here. She needs a haircut. Can you work her in?*

John: *She always shows up like this. If I don't take her she won't wait. Even if you talk her into waiting till Thursday, she may schedule the appointment but she'll go find someone else to cut it before then. Last time I didn't take her she went to another salon. And they didn't do a half bad job either. Just tell her to wait, I'll be able to take her in about twenty minutes.*

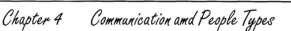

Margo   (returns to the reception desk): *OK, Katrina. He'll be with you in about twenty minutes.*

Katrina: *Wonderful. I guess I got here at just the right time. Does anyone have time to give me a manicure?*

Margo: *Stacie has some time right now. I'll page her.*

Katrina: *This is my lucky day.*

(Later, John has consulted with Katrina and is in the middle of her cut.)

Katrina: *John, do you think I should go a little shorter?*

John: *Why would you want that, Katrina. This is a perfect length.*

Katrina: *Because it's so flat. Maybe I should get a perm. Would you have time to perm my hair today?*

John: *A perm would probably help you get more lift. I'd be really careful, though, if I were you. Remember, your hair is tinted. What about getting just a root perm?*

Katrina: *Wow. You have some great solutions! Let's do it now!*

John: *Let me finish your cut and then I'll check to see if Robert can wrap your perm. If he can't do it, I'll find someone else.*

Since spontaneous characters are impulsive and like change, they can be fun as well as challenging. Develop rapport with them by being flexible and open minded, and then you can join the fun.

The Nurturing Personality

The nurturing personalities are driven by duty, responsibility, service, and belonging. They are thoughtful caregivers who bring gifts and unexpected pleasantries for no reason at all. Nurturers are sympathetic and helpful as co-workers. They care about customers and demonstrate a willingness to help customers in difficult situations. Sometimes the nurturer rescues others when the other person doesn't really need help.

Janet is on the phone in the break room speaking to her fiancé when Suzanne walks in and listens to the conversation.

Nurturing personalities are driven by duty, responsibility, service, and belonging.

Janet: OK. OK. I'll do it your mother's way. Bye. I'll see you tonight.

Suzanne: *That future mother-in-law of yours trying to run your wedding again?*

Janet: *Yeah. She is driving me crazy. She says we have to serve these strange-looking appetizers at the reception. I really don't want to, but I guess I better not make her angry.*

Suzanne: *You and your guy had better have a talk about his mother. This is no way for you to start a marriage. Would you like some potato soup? It's homemade.*

Janet: *No thanks, Suzanne. My appetite is gone now.*

Suzanne: *Honey, you are really having a tough time, aren't you? I'm telling you now, Janet. Take care of that mother-in law situation right now or you'll be sorry.*

Janet: *Suzanne, I know what I'm getting into. I'll handle it my own way.*

The Accommodating Personality

The accommodating personality is easy going and flexible. As a client, he can be indecisive, not wanting to commit himself and be dependent on a professional opinion. At his best he is the easiest client to service, and at his worst he is frustratingly slow at making up his mind. To work with him best, give him choices or, even better, yes or no closed questions rather than questions that require an open answer.

The primary disadvantage of indecisive clients is that they use up their service time trying to decide what they need or want. On the phone, they can be frustrating to the receptionist, and in the salon, they can make even the most patient salon professional lose her composure.

Carolyn: *Would you like to have a clear matte polish on your nails?*

Jerry: *I don't think so.*

Carolyn: *You'd like to have them buffed instead.*

Jerry: *Yes, if that's what you think I should do.*

Perhaps the most frustrating situation is when spontaneous and accommodating personalities come together in the same client. Salon professionals will need all the patience and perseverance they can muster to deal effectively with such clients.

Perhaps the most frustrating situation is when spontaneous and accomodating personalities come together in the same client.

Carl: *Hello there, Stacie. How is college going? Are you home for just the week end or do you have a few days off?*

Stacie: *I have a long weekend. No school Monday because of somebody's birthday or a holiday or something. I'm so glad to be home where you can do my color. It just isn't the same at school. Nobody there seems to know how to do my color right. Last time they did it it turned a funny purple color at the roots. Mom said I could get my hair red if you thought it was OK.*

Carl: *I thought you really liked that pastel blonde we have been doing. Are you sure you really want your hair red?*

Stacie: *Yeah, well maybe. What do you think?*

Carl: *I think you would look good in red hair; however, I have to tell you that if you decide on red you can't go back to pale blonde.*

Stacie: *Why can't you make it blonde again? I see all those super-models go from blonde to black to blonde again.*

Carl: *Because it would create too much damage. Your hair is already double processed. I'm afraid your hair might break.*

Stacie: *Oh . . . Well, I just don't know what to do.*

Carl: *You just have to remember that if you go red, you have to stay with either red or a darker color. You can't be pastel blonde for a long time, maybe a year.*

Stacie: *Ugh! Tell me what to do, Carl. I want it red, but I don't know if I'll like it.*

Carl: *Stacie, I can't decide for you. I have given you all the pros and cons, now you decide.*

Stacie: *Maybe I'll just get it permed instead.*

The Complaining Personality

Clients do us a favor when they complain; however, chronic complainers are so difficult to deal with that we have to be careful not to ignore their petty grievances. Complainers seem to enjoy misery, collecting and carrying it with them wherever they go. These are the people who must find fault with everything. If you say to them, "Isn't this an absolutely beautiful day?" the complainers retort, "Yes, but the sun is so bright it hurts my eyes."

As a co-worker, the complainer can be the dark side of the employee break room, leaching onto every opportunity to espouse his woes.

Carolyn: *Oh dear, what do I do next?*

John: *What's wrong, Carolyn?*

Carolyn: *Everything.*

John: *Everything?*

Carolyn: *Practically everything. I feel lousy. I think I'm coming down with something, and I have six clients left today.*

John: *I'm sure Diane would let you go home if you feel that bad.*

Carolyn: *Yes, but I have two nail fill clients that I know can't switch days.*

John: *Jennifer can do them. She is very good with sculptured nails.*

Carolyn: *Yes, but Judy, my six o'clock, would be furious. She doesn't like anyone but me doing her nails.*

John   (unsympathetically):   *Carolyn, if you were really sick you would go home.*

Carolyn: *OK, whatever you say.*

When the "poor me" personality of the complainer gets helpful suggestions, you may hear a few "Yes, but . . ." statements in return. Instead of helpful statements, try asking complainers what they think the solution might be.

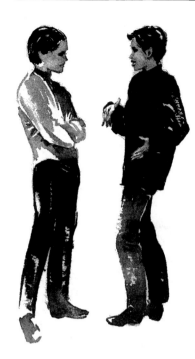

John: *I'm sure Diane would let you go home if you feel that bad.*

Carolyn: *Yes, but I have two nail fill clients that I know can't switch their days.*

John: *Well what do you think you should do then?*

Carolyn: *I could ask Jennifer to help. She is pretty good at sculptured nails. Judy, my six o'clock won't like it, but that's too bad. I've never canceled on her before, so she'll have to get over it. I'm going home.*

John: *Good decision, Carolyn.*

The Controlling Personality

The controlling personality knows all the answers. She is driven by knowledge, competency, and change and makes heavy demands on others. The controller can be manipulative, independent, and authoritative. When you see someone who isn't doing things right and you tell that person a better way to do it, you are being controlling. Controlling clients know how they want their services done. They demand service, attention, and quality.

Suzanne's client is getting her monthly facial.

Katy: *Suzanne, this steamer is too direct on my face. It isn't supposed to be this close, is it?*

Suzanne: *I'll move it back a little for you Katy. How's that?*

Katy: *That's better. You are going to custom blend my hydrating masque this time, aren't you?*

Suzanne: *Of course, I will. I always blend your masque.*

Katy: *Last time it didn't work as well. Are you sure you wrote down the right formula?*

Suzanne: *I'm sure I have the right formula. Let me read it to you. It's two parts creme, one part clay, three drops of hydration, and one half scoop of mud. Is that right?*

Katy: *That's right. Maybe you just didn't leave it on long enough.*

Suzanne: *I guess that's a possibility. I'll leave it on a few extra minutes this time.*

Challenging controlling clients when they are wrong will probably make them angry. Instead, guide them in the right direction so they have the opportunity to change their mind without losing their power.

The Compulsive Personality

Compulsion at its extreme is an obsession or an irresistible urge to act irrationally. Clients who are compulsive will brush nonexistent hair from your styling chair, demand that every hair be in the same place as the last time you cut their hair, and will stay with the same hairstyle forever if you let them.

Compulsive clients will resist change even when change is happening all around them. The key to changing a compulsive personality is to build trust slowly and guarantee your services (or products).

Carl feels that his client, Joan, should change her method of color. Her hair is graying rapidly around her hairline, and the highlighting process that Carl has used successfully for ten years is no longer camouflaging her gray.

Joan: *Maybe rather than using a different coloring process, you could just highlight it heavier. Wouldn't that cover the gray?*

Carl: *Joan, that would make it worse. Look closely at the gray around your hairline. There is almost no dark color left. It is all gray. Putting more highlighting there isn't going to help.*

Compulsive personalities are obsessive and sometimes act irrationally.

Joan: *It does look gray, doesn't it? But I'm really concerned about changing it. What did you want to do again?*

Carl: *There are several options. You could do all-over tinting; that would be more of a solid color than you have now. Or you could have some lowlighting; that's where I put some darker strands through the gray. That will just reduce the amount of gray that shows.*

Joan: *Tell you what, Carl. Do it the same as always this time and next time I'll try something different. OK?*

Carl: *All right, Joan. How about if I put some very small strands of darker color through the gray? If you let me do that today, I promise you will hardly even know it's there. It will be a beginning and then we can do just a little more each time. This way you won't see a major change.*

Joan: *As long as you promise that it won't be noticeable. Go ahead.*

The Amiable Personality

Amiable personalities are so comfortable with your salon that they might offer to answer the phone or help you clean up. They are the most loyal and forgiving of all client types, and at their best they will be your best public relations voice.

However, sometimes they will linger in the salon and talk even when you have other clients to service. The amiables are the personality types that can cross the line to your personal life and will be offended if you don't let them get close to you.

Monique's client, Peggy, has become too friendly. She wants Monique to go out with her and some friends to a nightclub on Friday. Monique does not want to go. There are several ways that Monique can handle the situation. She could go with Peggy, she could tell Peggy that she is busy or that salon policy prevents her from going out with a client. Monique could tell Peggy that she enjoys her very much as a client and does not want to jeopardize that stylist/client relationship. No matter which way Monique declines the offer, it will be difficult to sustain the amiable client's loyalty.

Peggy: *My hair looks great, as usual. Thanks, Monique.*

Monique: *I'm glad you like it, Peggy.*

Peggy: *Would you like to go to the Green Marble with me and a few friends on Friday night?*

Monique: *Oh, I don't think so Peggy.*

Peggy: *Oh, come on. It will be fun.*

Monique: *Well, for one thing, I have to work early Saturday so I don't usually go out on Fridays.*

Peggy: *But your favorite band, Morgo, is playing there. You can make an exception for one Friday night.*

Monique: *Peggy, I really enjoy cutting your hair and having time to talk to you. We always have a good time. However, I prefer not to mix my professional life with my personal one. I hope you understand.*

Peggy: *Sure, I guess I understand.*

Chapter Summary

1. Each of us makes judgments about others. Our body language and words will automatically indicate approval or disapproval of others, as judged by our life rules.

2. Unconditional positive regard to accept the many differences in other people's personalities, appearances, beliefs, intelligence, and decision-making processes without judgment. It does not mean you must agree with someone else's view, it simply means that you accept that they have a different set of life rules. To accept unconditional positive regard is to accept that people are different.

3. Life rules get passed along, generation to generation, and when they are challenged we feel insecure. Some life rules remain valid through adulthood and others become archaic as we mature.

4. People are more susceptible to anger and conflict when they hang onto archaic life rules without objectively studying their tapes in light of new information. We call such people "stuck in their ways."

5. The tone of your internal dialogue is a result of the kind of memory tapes that are created by your life rules. They can affect you positively or negatively. You can change your memory tapes by consciously replacing them with positive messages.

6. In a salon atmosphere, your personal space is invaded regularly and personalities often bump into each other. Because intimacy is the nature of the salon industry, it is imperative that salon professionals learn to communicate feelings as well as words and concepts.

7. By voicing petty grievances, communicating needs, and having realistic expectations of others, you can avoid collecting negative feelings.

8. Spontaneous personalities are driven by action and tend to be impulsive, happy go lucky, and cheerful. Because spontaneous personalities don't like to schedule in advance, they are more likely to call the day they want an appointment.

9. Clients with nurturing personalities are driven by duty, responsibility, service, and belonging. The accommodating personality is easy going and flexible, while complaining personalities need to find fault with everything. They seem to enjoy misery, collecting and carrying it with them wherever they go.

10. Controlling personalities think they know all the answers, and they make heavy demands for service, attention, and quality. On the other hand, amiable personalities enjoy a close relationship with their salon professionals and are therefore more forgiving.

Chapter 5

Gender Communication

*W*e think of language differences as typically cultural. However, in communicating with clients, understanding subtle language differences can make the difference between keeping clients and losing them. Every age group has it own unique communication rules. Words that help you communicate with children are different from the words you use to communicate with more mature clients. Similarly, skillfully conversing with a fifteen-year-old girl takes a whole different approach from consulting with a middle-aged businessperson.

To complicate matters, men and women communicate differently. In the cosmetology business, we have salon professionals who are both male and female and clients who are also male and female. Therefore, it is imperative to learn how to communicate with the opposite sex.

Communication differences between sexes and age groups exist in varying degrees or sometimes not at all. We are all primarily individuals with our own way of communicating, secondly male or female, and finally young or mature. This chapter presents tendencies, not universal truths.

Male and Female Communication

Historically, women have been taught to avoid confrontation. Women will use an indirect approach, such as asking a question to get what they want. They will say, "Don't you think we should spend more time together?" instead of saying, "I think that we should spend more time together." Men have more difficulty reading between the lines or reading body language and tend not to recognize indirect messages or nonverbal communication. If a woman says, "This is really heavy," a man might reply, "Yes it is," while another woman would interpret the sentence as a cry for help. A man expects to hear the specific words, "This is too heavy for me. Please help."

Men Like Solutions

Men tend to give solutions and invalidate feelings, while women offer unsolicited advice and directions. A male stylist might try to solve his client's personal problems when she voices them and consequently alienates his client. She just wants to talk and doesn't need him to fix her problem.

Women will use an indirect approach, such as asking a question to get what they want. Men have more difficulty reading between the lines or reading body language and tend not to recognize indirect messages or nonverbal communication.

Sarah: *I'm sorry I had to reschedule my appointment, Carl. I have had the most frustrating experience with my doctor. I had an appointment for an exam last Thursday morning, the day I was supposed to get my color. I sat in the reception room for an hour and then in the exam room for twenty minutes before the nurse came in and told me the doctor was still at the hospital. I missed my appointment with you, I was late picking up my daughter from nursery school, and I got a parking ticket. I am really ticked off that I have to go back again for my appointment.*

Carl: *I hear you, Sarah. You don't deserve to be treated that way. There are lots of good doctors out there. Find another one.*

Sarah: *I probably should. That doctor can be so condescending sometimes. He talks like I'm an idiot when it comes to my own body.*

Carl: *You're an intelligent woman, Sarah. You don't have to put up with that patronizing attitude. Doctors these days are beginning to realize that they have to treat their patients with respect and consideration. Sarah, you need to find another doctor.*

Sarah   (feels she has to justify her choice of doctors to Carl): *I can't find another doctor just like that. He knows my medical history, and my kids like him. My husband Tom isn't crazy about him, though. Tom hates to wait.*

Carl: *Oh Sarah, Sarah. I'm telling you. Find another doctor. I'll get some referrals for you.*

Sarah   (becomes even more irritated with Carl): *Carl, can't you just listen without telling me what to do? I know I could find a new doctor, but I have confidence in the one I have. I'm just having a problem with him right now.*

Carl: *I apologize, Sarah. I thought you were asking for help.*

Women Like Sharing

When a woman shares a problem, she wants empathy and may or may not want solutions to her problem. She needs to know that others understand the frustration or pain she is going through.

When men express a problem, it is with the intention of finding a solution. Imagine the frustration of a man wanting a solution and a woman offering empathy instead, or a woman needing understanding of a situation and a man giving her a lecture on solving the problem. Men need to realize that when a woman is upset she has little ability to appreciate solutions. What she needs is to be heard. Offering solutions will alienate her and could increase her anger.

Janet and Robert are in the break room having lunch. It has been a slow day in the salon.

Janet: *I just can't stand this place any longer. I don't feel like I'm learning anything. I feel like I'm going to be an assistant forever. All I do is clean up after everybody. It's really getting to me. And business has been so . . . slow lately. I'm afraid that when I do start getting my own clients, there won't be enough for me to make decent money.*

Robert: *Well, why don't you just find another job if you don't like it here?*

Janet (slightly perturbed): *Oh, Robert. Don't get radical on me, I don't want to quit. I just need to complain. Can't I just complain a little?*

Robert: *Sure, Janet. Complain all you want.*

Women Tend to Read between the Lines

Likewise, a female stylist can interpret a male client's comment incorrectly. Because women like to read between the lines, they can create a problem where there isn't one.

Jennifer: *Good morning, Mr. Crowley. It's nice to see you again.*

Mr. Crowley: *Thank you, Jennifer. I really liked the haircut you gave me last month. The only problem I had was when this piece in the back sticks up.*

Jennifer: *It's frustrating when you have a bad hair day. Isn't it strange that something so trivial can start your whole day off bad? I'm sorry you had a problem with your cut. Perhaps I can change the angle of the cut so that it will lay down better. Would you like to have this back piece a little longer?*

Mr. Crowley: *I just want to know what to do when it sticks up.*

Jennifer: *That is what I am trying to do.*

Mr. Crowley: *No. The cut you did was just fine. When you styled my hair it looked great. I want to know how you did it.*

Jennifer: *Oh! You want some of the styling gel I used.*

How Ugly Will I Look?

When a client wants to grow his or her hair out a little longer, uppermost in the male mind is "How long will it take?", while the female mind focuses on "How painful will it be?" or "How ugly will I look?"

Phyllis is a middle-aged woman who has been a salon client for many years. She has decided to grow her hair longer because, as she put it, "I want to feel hair on my shoulders one more time before I'm too old for long hair." Notice the way Janet expresses empathy for Phyllis as compared to the words Carl uses.

Janet: *Hello, Phyllis. Please come with me and I will get you prepared for your perm. I see your hair is longer than you used to wear it.*

Phyllis: *I'm growing it out. What can I do with it as it grows longer? I know it will get into that awkward stage when it doesn't look good no matter what I do.*

Janet: *It can certainly be a painful process, especially if you want to grow all the layers out. I remember when I grew mine out. I felt like wearing a bag over my head for six months. I'm sure Carl will consult with you about it.*

Phyllis: *Good, maybe he'll have some ideas.*
        (Janet prepares Phyllis for her perm.)

Carl: *Phyllis, your hair is certainly getting longer. Aren't you pleased?*

Phyllis: *Yes, but this growing out business is really hard. It's taking forever! What can I do with it while it's growing?*

Carl: *Your hair grows about half an inch a month, so it will take about eight months to grow it to the length you want.*

Phyllis: *Are you saying I'm going to be ugly for eight months? What do I do with this mess in the mean time?*

Carl: *Phyllis, Phyllis, Phyllis, it will be just fine. Don't worry. If it doesn't work, you can cut it short again.*

Phyllis   (becoming irritated with Carl):   *Carl, I'm growing it out. I don't plan to cut it off, so why don't you just do something so that it looks good at this length?*

Because women like to read between the lines, they can create a problem where there isn't one.

Carl: *OK, Phyllis, there are several options. You might think about getting a softer perm so your layers don't get too bushy. You'll also have to spend a little more time in the morning to style your hair till it grows a little more.*

Phyllis: *So you're saying that all I have to do is take a little extra time with it?*

Carl: *Basically, yes.*

Phyllis: *OK. I can do that.*

You Shouldn't Worry So Much

There are a few male sayings that can invalidate a woman's feelings. For example, telling a client she shouldn't worry so much could stimulate feelings of anger and resentment or a sense of inadequacy.

There are a few male sayings that can invalidate a woman's feelings.

Cindy is a young mother of three. Since the birth of her youngest last year, she has noticed an increasing number of gray hairs appearing. Last month at a family gathering, her mother remarked that Cindy was getting prematurely gray. Today Cindy has an appointment for her regular haircut and wants to talk to her stylist, John, about haircolor.

Cindy: *My mother says I'm getting gray just like her. I can't stand it. I'm only thirty-two and I don't want gray hair yet, but I'm afraid to color my hair. What can I do?*

John: *You shouldn't be so concerned about a few gray hairs, Cindy. You don't have nearly enough gray hair to begin thinking about permanent color.*

Cindy: *But then how can I get rid of them? I have some friends who color their hair and it looks so colored. You know, red and dry looking. I don't want that.*

John: *Leave it alone, Cindy. You can only see ten or fifteen in the front area. Don't worry about it. Wait till you get more gray before you put color on it.*

Cindy (exasperated): *John, I don't want gray hair. I don't want even one gray hair. Don't you understand? I want it my natural color. I don't want anyone to know my hair has color in it. Can you do it or not?*

It's Not Such a Big Deal

When a man says "it's not such a big deal," a woman thinks he is saying that her concerns are trivial.

Marc's client is Lynne, a new mother who is upset about hair loss. Marc is familiar with this problem and doesn't seem concerned at all.

Lynne: *Marc, I'm losing a lot of hair recently. Every day the drain is full of hair after my shower. Does it look like something is wrong with my scalp?*

Marc: *Lynne, how old is your baby?*

Lynne: *She is almost four months old. Why?*

Marc: *It is very common for women to lose some hair three or four months after childbirth. Most women lose it mostly around their hairline. It's not a big deal.*

Lynne: *It's a big deal to me. My hair's falling out. How much am I going to lose?*

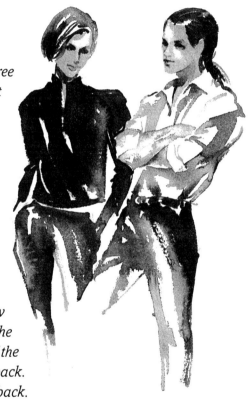

Marc: *It's hard to tell. In some women the hair loss is noticeable. In others, you can't tell at all.*

Lynne: *Now you really have me upset. My hair is thin enough already. Is it gone forever, can I stop it? Will it grow back or what?*

Marc: *Your hair really is thin, isn't it? But it will grow back. It takes a while, but it grows back. Look at the bright side. See John working on the other side of the salon? His hair is thinning and his won't grow back. Yours could take a year or more, but it will grow back.*

Lynne (now deeply depressed): *Well Marc, I don't want to hear any more. I think I'd rather not know anything else. Just get my hair cut so I can go home.*

I Got It! This Is What You Should Do

A male tendency is to solve problems. To a female, sharing problems is a way to think out loud or ask for comfort. She doesn't necessarily need to have her problem solved.

Monique and John are in the break room having lunch.

Monique: *Mary Lou is on my book again today. I just cut her hair last week. She never likes it the first time I cut it. She's always back in a few days needing the front shorter or the back thinner or something. She really upsets me. Have you ever watched her?*

John: *No. I don't think so. Is she the client who brings the two small boys?*

Monique: *Yes, the two that fight all the time. That's her. She grabs a piece of hair in her fingers and tells me to cut it. She whines and complains about the way I do her hair. I just don't need clients like her.*

John: *This is what you should do next time. Just tell her that you think another stylist would do a better job. Refer her to Jennifer. That would solve your problem.*

Monique: *No, I'm not going to refer her to Jennifer. I'll handle it myself. I really don't need you to tell me what to do.*

John: *Sorry, I didn't mean to stir you up. I thought you wanted to solve a problem.*

Almost everyone is annoyed by someone who nags, and men seem to be especially irritated by unsolicited advice or harmless criticism.

Unsolicited Advice

Almost everyone is annoyed by someone who nags, and men seem to be especially irritated by unsolicited advice or harmless criticism. When a woman says, "Your station is a mess, you should clean it up," it translates as nagging to the man and reminding to the woman.

Diane: *Robert, you never remember to empty the trash in the facial room. This place is always a mess. I just can't stand it.*

Robert: *I'm sorry if I am not doing my job. That's what it sounds like you are saying, anyway. I have forgotten to empty the trash a few times; however, most of the time I remember.*

Diane: *I apologize, Robert. Yes, you do a great job. It's just that sometimes you forget the trash. Please try to remember next time.*

In another situation, Suzanne, the esthetician, walks into the break room when Carl is having lunch.

Suzanne: *Carl, that pizza is full of fat. Don't you know it is bad for your heart?*

Carl: *Suzanne, I very seldom eat high-fat foods. I'm not stupid, you know. I am well aware of the food I put into my body and what it does to me, and I don't need your advice.*

Suzanne: *Sorry, Carl. I didn't mean anything by it.*

Questions or Objections

Our society teaches women to avoid confrontation; therefore, to express an opinion or an objection, women will often offer a question instead of a direct statement.

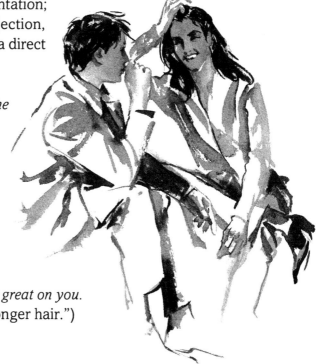

Female client Roxanne: *Don't you think the color is a little dark?*

Carl: *No, it's perfect.*
(What the client wants to hear from her stylist: "It looks dark to you, doesn't it?")

Female client Cathy: *Do you really think I should grow out the back of my hair?*

John: *Sure. It's the style, and it would be great on you.*
(What she is saying: "I don't want to have longer hair.")

Small Talk or Big Talk

Many women use small talk as a vehicle to connect with another person. Talking about personal topics such as relationships and feelings is a way for women to build rapport with another person.

Male clients may view small talk as a waste of time. They view talking as an exchange of information that leads to solving an issue. Their topics of conversation are often centered around facts about sports, news, or business issues.

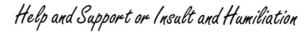

Help and Support or Insult and Humiliation

Women like to share their misfortunes and find support and camaraderie comforting. They feel that sharing creates a rapport with others. Men think that sharing troubles is the same as sharing humiliation. Because men seek respect, approval, and self-sufficiency, sharing problems with anyone other than very close friends is an admission that they are not in control of their lives. Needing help is a sign of weakness to men, and they need to feel self-sufficient. Women kindly offer sympathy to men to support them; however, sympathetic comments can humiliate a man.

Janet: *Hi, Dave. Sorry to hear about you losing your job. You must feel terrible. You were with that company for at least twenty years, weren't you?*

Dave: *Yeah, I was.*

Janet: *That was really unfair of them to do that to you. You must be devastated!*

Dave   (the pitch of his voice becomes higher and his words are clipped short):   *Yes, Janet. It is upsetting; however, I think I can handle it.*

Janet gets the message that Dave doesn't want to talk about it.

Opinions and Decisions

Women ask for opinions to be sure they are considering all aspects of a situation. They may or may not use those opinions. Men are inclined not to ask for opinions, and when they are queried for opinions, they consider it wasted effort when their opinion is not used. In decision making, women want consensus, while men prefer dictating and not wasting time with discussions of everybody's feelings.

Perhaps it seems impossible for men and women to speak the same language. The following are some guidelines to help you break down that communication barrier.

- Men need to listen for feelings rather than offer immediate solutions to women's problems. Women need to become more solution-oriented when a man offers a problem.

- Women can try to accept men's words at face value rather than reading covert messages into a man's words. Men need to learn that meta-messages are as powerful as the words themselves.

- Men don't want unsolicited advice; they interpret it as nagging.

- Often women object to a situation by asking questions, while men tend to make direct objections.

- Sometimes men need to learn that small talk can build rapport with others. Women need to learn when to end the small talk and get down to business.

- Sympathetic comments to a man can humiliate him, while the same comment to a woman would be interpreted as a caring response.

Women ask for opinions to be sure they are considering all aspects of a situation. Men are inclined not to ask for opinions, they consider it wasted effort when their opinion is not used.

Children and Teen Dialogue

Working with small children can be fun for some stylists and a nightmare for others. Stylists who enjoy small children often have a natural ability to captivate kids' attention. Small children are mother directed. When they find themselves in unfamiliar surroundings, they need to have mom close at hand for support. After a few positive visits to the salon, those same clinging children transform themselves into extroverted miniature clients with their own ideas about how they want to look. Ages two to five can be the most challenging children's age group. To keep children in that age group as still as possible, direct their attention from the project at hand. Give them something unfamiliar to touch and play with, such as a brush, a clippie, or an unbreakable mirror.

If it is the child's first haircut, he might be frightened that cutting his hair might hurt, like cutting his finger. Children can also be afraid that you might cut their skin with your shears or clippers. Since blow dryer noise can also be frightening, you could let them handle the dryer first and demonstrate its harmlessness by aiming it at your arm first. The more they know, the better they will be.

As children grow older, they begin to develop a relationship with their hairdresser. It is common for them to grow so attached that they are perhaps even more loyal than their parents.

Monique: *Why it's Joey! I thought you moved away. It's great to see you again. How are you?*

Joey: *Hi, Monique. I came back to get a haircut.*

Monique: *You mean you came all the way from Indiana to get a haircut? Did you miss me that much, Joey?*

Joey: (blushes): *I just like the way you cut my hair. I got it cut at a new place, but they didn't do it the same. I want it done the way you used to do it.*

Joey's mom: *Actually, we came back for a wedding and decided to give Joey a treat. He really misses you cutting his hair.*

After a few positive visits to the salon, some children transform themselves into extroverted miniature clients with their own ideas about how they want to look.

When children are small they take direction from adults fairly easily. However, as they grow they have their own ideas about what they like and dislike. Sometimes the child has his idea of a haircut and the parent has another, leaving the salon professional in the middle of the struggle.

A similar situation occurred at the Sensations Salon, with Robert and his twelve-year-old client.

Margo: *Good morning, Sensations Salon, this is Margo. How can I help you?*

Nancy: *Hi, Margo. This is Nancy Pettey. My son, Brad, is coming in for a haircut today. I need to talk to Robert about how I want Brad's hair cut.*

Margo: *Hold on just a minute, Nancy. Robert is on break. Let me page him for you.*

Robert: *Hello, this is Robert.*

Nancy: *This is Nancy Pettey, Brad's mom.*

Robert: *Oh hello, Nancy. What can I do for you?*

Nancy: *Robert, you are cutting Brad's hair this afternoon and I want you to cut that front piece of hair off.*

Robert: *He has been growing that long for months. You mean he wants to cut it off now?*

Nancy: *No. That's the point. He wants it long and I want it short and that's why I'm calling you. I want it off!*

Robert: *I can't just cut it off, Nancy.*

Nancy: *Robert, I'm the person who pays for the haircut so I want it cut the way I like it. OK.*

Robert: *I can't just cut it off. However, I can talk to him about changing his style. I realize that you pay for his haircuts; however, when he is sitting in my chair, he is my client. I can't, in good conscience, cut his hair off without his permission. Maybe you should talk to him before he gets here; you know, get some kind of agreement with him.*

(Nancy is very quiet and Robert doesn't know what to do.)

Robert: *Nancy, are you still there?*

Nancy: *Yes, Robert. I'm here.*

Robert: *I can discuss changing his style, but I can't promise you he will agree to cut off the hair that he has waited for so long. That is about the best I can do. By the way, what don't you like about his hair right now?*

Nancy: *The way it falls across his eyes all the time. He is constantly pushing it aside.*

Robert: *If I could get his hair out of his face without cutting it, would that satisfy you?*

Nancy: *Well, I don't see how you could do that but, yes, that would be all right.*

Robert: *Great. I'll do my best to get Brad's hair out of his eyes.*

Nancy: *Thank you, Robert.*

Teen Talk

For the most part, adult clients have enough experience in salons to be able to communicate in the language of hairdressing. When you say *layering, acid wave,* or *nail balancing,* adult clients will have a reasonably good understanding of the terms. Teens, however, have their own terms for hair, and because teens are loyal once they learn to trust, it is worth the investment in time and effort to learn their language. When speaking to a teen with specific ideas about how she would like her hair to look, be sure to listen carefully and watch her body language.

John: *Hello, Megan. My name is John and I am going to style your hair today. This is your first time here. How do you feel about going to a new hairdresser?*

Megan: *I don't like anyone new unless I know they can do it or if they have a picture or something to go by. I wouldn't trust them; my hair means too much me.*

John: *I'm glad you're honest with me, Megan. I'd like to consult with you before we do anything. How would you like to have your hair cut?*

Megan: *I want bangs but no bangs, long bangs I mean that go toward my face, but not very many, you know. Just this piece cut to here and then this piece cut to here and then maybe one in the middle on this side.*

John: *Would a picture of a similar cut help you describe what you want?*

Megan: *Yes. Then you would know exactly what to do.*

John (gets several styling books and opens one to a photograph): *How is this picture?*

Megan: *Yeah, see the pieces she has that go toward her face. That's what I want except I don't want it so pouffy on top.*

John: *You mean you want definite pieces cut on the side that don't blend into the rest of your haircut?*

Megan: *Yeah, I think you have it.*

Teens have their own terms for hair, and because teens are loyal once they learn to trust, it is worth the investment in time and effort to learn their language.

Selling Retail

Teens, just like adults, are attracted to products that look and smell good. However, teens are more likely to switch brands if a new product looks tempting and are less likely to stick with a *unique* are key words when selling to teens.

Teens and Haircolor

Carl: *Hello, Megan. I see on my schedule that you are here to have your hair highlighted. It looks like you have had it highlighted before.*

Megan: *I had it highlighted last year at spring break right before I went to Florida on vacation. See how light it is on the ends? I want it to look like that all over.*

Carl: *Megan, you want the dark area on top to match the blonde on the bottom?*

Megan: *Kinda, only I want more blonde on the top. I want it white like it used to be when I was a kid.*

Carl: *If I do a heavy weave highlight to make your hair that light, then in a few months you will have definite new growth. In other words, you'll have light brown roots.*

Megan: *It's OK. I'll get it touched up when I need it. If I decide it's too much trouble to keep it blonde, then I'll have some brown put back in it.*

Carl: *Do you want your hair streaked with pale blonde or do you want it to be all over colored?*

Megan: *I want it all blonde. I want it almost white like the ends of my hair.*

Carl: *That's a big commitment, Megan. You will have to have your new growth done every four weeks. If you get some pale blonde streaks instead, you will be much blonder than you are right now, it will look more natural, and it won't have to be done as often.*

Megan: *That's OK. It doesn't have to look natural. It just has to look good.*

Carl: *OK then. We'll make you a blonde. No matter which way you go, you'll have to be sure to get the right shampoos and conditioners to take care of your long hair.*

Teens and Perming

Carl: *Hello, Kristie. I have seen you in the salon getting haircuts before and I have permed your mother's hair, but this is the first time I have met you. Have you ever had a perm before?*

Kristie: *Yes, I had it permed here before.*

Carl: *When was that?*

Kristie: *In seventh grade—about four years ago.*

Carl: *Did you like it?*

Kristie: *Yeah, but it fell out the first time and I had to do it again.*

Carl: *Did it hold the second time?*

Kristie: *Yeah, it did. I really liked it. I could dry it straight or leave it curly.*

Carl: *Was your hair as long then as it is now?*

Kristie: *Nuh uh, it only went to my shoulders. Here is a picture of me with it permed.*

Carl: *Great. I'm glad you thought of bringing a picture. Your hair is much longer now. Do you want as much wave as last time?*

Kristie: *What I want this time is to have it a lot curlier. I want it curly all the way up.*

Carl: *Then you must want some layering.*

Kristie: *You mean I have to have layers to get this kind of curl?*

Carl: *Yes. If you leave it one length, no matter how curly we make it, your hair will hang in waves instead of curls. It has to have many layers to create that kind of loose curly look. Your only other option is to get it permed one length and then set your hair to get the type of curl you want.*

Today's senior clients are healthier and more active than senior clients of the past. Because of strides in medicine and health management, there are many more elderly than there were just a decade ago. Old people aren't as "old" anymore. They stay active, pay attention to their bodies, and want to look good, too. Today it is common for a seventy-year-old client to wear current hairstyles and dress fashionably. Most salons have at least a few senior clients, and pleasing them can be slightly different from pleasing other age groups.

Don't patronize clients because they are elderly, even though you must understand their special needs. Mature clients are often more physically compromised; they walk and move more slowly. Elderly clients are more susceptible to sudden health changes, which means changes in medications. They are more likely to have hearing loss and poor eyesight than younger clients, and because their immune system loses its ability as they age, seniors are more likely to get fungus infections in their nails or develop scalp disorders.

Most salons have at least a few senior clients, and pleasing them can be slightly different from pleasing other age groups.

Diane, the salon manager, is at the reception desk placing a supply order when her next client, Helen, walks in carrying a carefully wrapped rose. Helen is seventy-seven-years old and has been Diane's client for sixteen years. She has a standing appointment every Friday at 10:00 A.M.

Diane: *Oh, hi there, Helen. I'll be right with you, I just have to call in an order first.*

Helen: *Take your time, take your time. I'll just get some coffee while I wait. I brought you one of my husband's prize roses. Do you have a vase to put it in?*

Margo: *That is a beautiful rose, Helen. Give it to me and I'll put it in some water. Go ahead and get your coffee. Diane will be right with you.*

(Helen pours herself coffee and walks to Diane's styling chair.)

Diane: *OK. I'm all done. How are you, Helen? How did your hair hold up this week?*

Helen: *Not so well. I just don't know what's wrong. You just gave me a perm two weeks ago. My hair is really dry, too. Did you use the same perm?*

(Diane picks up a hairbrush and examines Helen's hair closely.)

Diane: *Yes, Helen, I did. And the same perm rods and the same process time. It just doesn't feel like your hair anymore. Is your skin also dry?*

Helen: *Come to think of it, yes. It is drier than ever before. I notice it mostly on my arms. The skin is really flaky.*

Diane: *Have you started taking any new medicine or changed your diet?*

Helen: *I started taking a new medication about a month ago. It's a diuretic to get rid of the swelling I have in my ankles. It worked a miracle. My ankles aren't swollen a bit now. Do you think that medicine could affect my hair?*

Diane: *Of course it could, Helen. Doesn't it make sense that a medication that removes water from your system would also take moisture from your skin and hair?*

Helen: *What can you do about it?*

Diane: *What I can do is give you an intensive hair and scalp treatment. However, if I were you I would talk to my doctor about the dryness. Maybe she could adjust the medication or something.*

Helen: *You're probably right, Diane. I'll check with my doctor. I have to see her soon anyway. Will this treatment fix my hair?*

Diane: *It will help tremendously and it will last through a few shampoos. I think it would be a good idea to do treatments on you every two weeks for a while as long as you are taking that diuretic. The treatments are fifteen dollars.*

Helen: *That could get expensive, Diane. Isn't there a rinse that would help?*

Diane: *Your hair needs more than a simple creme rinse. Besides, all they do is make hair like yours limp. Then you would have dry, limp hair. A treatment puts essential nutrients back into your hair. It will make it feel like new hair again. You can save money if you buy a series. If you buy five treatments, you can get the sixth one free. How does that sound?*

Helen: *Diane, that's still expensive for me. I just don't know if I can afford to spend that much money on my hair.*

Diane: *I understand, Helen. How about if I do one treatment today at the regular price? Then next week you can tell me if it is worth getting more. If you still want to buy the series, I'll let you pay the balance of the five treatments next week. How does that sound?*

Helen: *So what you are saying is that I pay fifteen dollars today and if I like it I can pay the additional sixty dollars next week? I'll still get the sixth one free?*

Diane: *Yes, that's right. You'll still get the sixth one free. Shall we go ahead with the treatment today?*

Helen: *OK. Let's do it.*
(A week later Helen arrives for her standing appointment.)

Diane: *Helen, how did your hair hold up this week?*

Helen: *Diane, it was wonderful. It stayed in all week. And feel it— it still feels good.*

Diane: *So you liked that treatment?*

Helen: *I have to admit, it did work, didn't it?*

Diane: *So do you think you want to continue with the series?*

Helen: *Yes, I think it would be a good idea, Diane.*

Janet is assisting Carl by applying color to a senior client's new growth. Mrs. Henderson, the client, is cringing every time Janet touches the color brush to her head. Carl, working in the next chair, notices Mrs. Henderson's discomfort.

Carl: *Are you OK, Mrs. Henderson? It looks like you are in pain.*

Mrs. Henderson: *Carl, it never hurts like this when you put my color on. Can she be a little more gentle?*

Janet: *Sorry, ma'am. I guess I'm a little heavy handed.*

Mrs. Henderson:	*It feels like you are stabbing me with that brush. Can't you find one with softer bristles?*
Carl:	*Go easy there, Janet. Mrs. Henderson has a sensitive scalp. And be sure to put creme around her hairline before you apply color there or you'll never get the stains off. She is allergic to the stain remover.*

(Janet changes the angle of her brush application and uses gentler strokes to apply the color.)

Janet:	*Is this better, Mrs. Henderson?*
Mrs. Henderson:	*Yes, sweetie. That's much better.*

Mature clients tend to become realistic about hair expectations. By now they know that fine, thin hair will never look thick and luxurious. However, acceptance of self and limitations doesn't mean that they will accept less than good service. No matter if your client has worn her hair the same away for thirty years and doesn't want it changed or if she likes to wear different looks every season: She still shouldn't be taken for granted.

Always consult with senior clients before performing a nail service. For those clients who are susceptible to fungus infections, suggest that they purchase, from you, their own implements for you to use on them for their service. Many nail companies now provide a packet of implements for you to retail. Many clients, not just seniors, appreciate the option of purchasing their own sanitized manicuring tools.

Carolyn, the salon nail technician, is giving Mrs. Henderson a manicure while her color is processing.

Carolyn:	*Hello, Mrs. Henderson, it's nice to see you again. Has it been a whole month since your last manicure? Let me look at your hands.*

Mrs. Henderson:	*Hi, Carolyn. Yes, it has been a long time. I don't mean to go so long between manicures, but I get so busy I don't have time. Look at my ring finger. The nail looks a little strange. Does that look like a fungus infection?*
Carolyn:	*Let me see. I don't think so. It looks more like a bruise to me. This doesn't look anything like the fungus you had when you first started coming here. Just in case, do you still have any of that cream your doctor gave you last time?*
Mrs. Henderson:	*Last time I'm sure I got that fungus when I had a manicure at that other salon. I can't get it here because I have my own manicure packet. Right? You don't use my stuff on anyone else, do you?*
Carolyn:	*Of course not, Mrs. Henderson. I keep it locked up in my cabinet with your name on it. Everytime you get a manicure I sterilize your tools, seal them in a zip bag, and lock them away. There is no way you can catch anything here.*
Mrs. Henderson:	*Well, I'll trust that you are being honest with me. You think it looks like a bruise?*
Carolyn:	*Yeah. It looks like you shut your finger in a drawer or something.*
Mrs. Henderson	(begins to get irritated with Carolyn): *Well, I'm not so old that I wouldn't remember shutting my finger in a drawer, would I?*
Carolyn:	*Yes, Mrs. Henderson. I didn't mean to get you upset. It just looks like a bruise to me. I know there are times when I have a bruise that I can't account for. Sometimes I just get in a hurry and bump into something without realizing it. I thought that might happen to you, too.*
Mrs. Henderson:	*Uhm . . . I suppose that could happen, but I'm still going to have a doctor check it out.*
Carolyn:	*I think that is a very good idea. Then you will know for sure. Would you like to have an herbology treatment today?*

Mature clients tend to become realistic about hair expectations. However, acceptance of self and limitations doesn't mean that they will accept less than good service.

Mrs. Henderson:	*I don't think I have time for it. I'm getting a pedicure as soon as I'm finished here.*
Carolyn:	*Yes. I'm doing your pedicure also.*
Mrs. Henderson:	*I thought Suzanne was doing my pedicure. I don't like it when you people switch on me like that. Shouldn't you let me know when things change like that? Where is Suzanne today, anyway?*
Carolyn:	*She had a family emergency and had to leave just a few minutes ago. I hope you don't mind if I do your pedicure.*
Mrs. Henderson:	*I suppose it's OK. Although Suzanne has been working on getting rid of the callous on the ball of my foot. Do you know how to do that?*
Carolyn:	*I do a lot of pedicures, and many of my clients have the same problem. I really enjoy pedicuring, I think even more than manicuring.*
Mrs. Henderson:	*Is that so? It's certainly nice to know that there is someone else besides Suzanne who can take care of my feet.*

Chapter Summary

1. To communicate with clients, we must understand the subtle language differences that can make the difference between keeping clients and losing them.

2. Communication differences between sexes and age groups exist in varying degrees or sometimes not at all. We are all primarily individuals with our own ways of communicating, secondly male or female, and finally young or mature.

3. Male-female communication can be difficult for many reasons. In their process of "helping" women, men tend to invalidate women's feelings. When women think they are "helping" men, men think women are nagging.

4. Men have more difficulty reading between the lines or reading body language than women and tend not to recognize

indirect messages or nonverbal communication. Women have difficulty accepting men's words at face value.

5. Men think small talk is a waste of time, while women use it as a way of building rapport with others.

6. Patience and understanding are a must for stylists who style small children. When children find themselves in unfamiliar surroundings, they need to have mom close at hand for support. After a few positive visits to the salon, those same clinging children transform themselves into extroverted miniature clients with their own ideas about how they want to look.

7. As children grow into adolescence, they begin to challenge their parents' views of how they should look.

8. The language of teenagers can seem like speaking in a foreign language. They have their own terms for hair, and because teens are loyal, once they learn to trust, it is worth the investment in time and effort to learn their language. When speaking to a teen with specific ideas about how she would like her hair to look, be sure to listen carefully and watch her body language.

9. Because of strides in medicine and health management, there are many more elderly than there were just a decade ago. Today it is common for a seventy-year-old client to wear current hairstyles and dress fashionably. Most salons have at least a few senior clients, and pleasing them can be slightly different from pleasing other age groups.

10. Mature clients might have a more difficult time fitting into the shampoo bowl. In addition, their scalps are often more sensitive to temperature changes. Skin can get thinner, become almost transparent, and become more sensitive to chemical services.

The Salon Phone

Margo: *Good afternoon, Sensations Salon, this is Margo. How can I help you?*

Caller 1: *This is Sherice. I need to make an appointment with Janet.*

Margo: *Could you hold please while I get the next line?*

Caller 1: *Yes, I can hold.*

Margo: *Thank you. (Margo switches to the next ringing line.) Good afternoon, Sensations Salon, this is Margo. Could you hold please?*

Caller 2: *This is long distance.*

Margo: *I could call you right back.*

Caller 2: *No, I'll wait.*

Margo: *I'll be just a second while I put the next caller on hold and schedule my first caller.*

Caller 2: *OK.*

Margo: *Good afternoon, Sensations Salon, this is Margo. Could you hold please?*

Caller 3: *Sure.*

Margo (goes back to Caller 1): *Sherice, I have a long-distance call. Can you hold a little longer?*

Caller 1: *No problem.*

Margo: *Thanks, Sherice.*

Margo (switched to Caller 2): *How may I help you?*

Caller 2: *I need to change an appointment I have with Suzanne. It is on Tuesday the 2nd and I need to make it on the following Tuesday, the 9th.*

Margo: *Your name please?*

Caller 2: *This is Penny Jackson.*

Margo: *That will work just fine, Penny. Same time a week later, OK?*

Caller 2: *Great, I'll see you then. Bye.*

Margo: *Thank you, Penny. Good bye.* (Margo goes to Caller 3). *This is Margo, could you hold just a little longer?*

Caller 3: *This is Marc's sister. Just tell him to call me later.*

Margo: *OK. I'll give him the message. Good bye.* (Back to caller 1). *Sorry to keep you waiting, Sherice. How can I help you?*

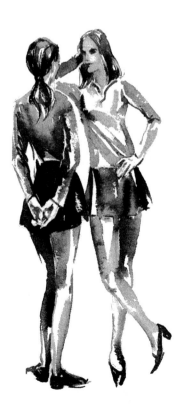

The telephone is probably the world's most powerful communication tool. Now that cellular phones have grown smaller and more affordable, we can carry a phone with us anywhere. It is possible now never to be unreachable. Since an increasing percentage of our communication with clients takes place over the phone, it is important for us to develop good telephone skills.

Remember that 55% of the message a client gets from us is in visual cues (body language and gestures). When you are speaking to a client on the phone, that person cannot see your body language. Miscommunication is easy because the client can only imagine (with her ears) what your body language is saying.

In most salons, every staff member will, at some time or another, have to answer the phone or make phone calls to clients. In this chapter, the term *receptionist* refers to any salon professional who happens to be on the phone. In addition, much of the information about customer service is as applicable in person as it is on the phone.

Smiling on the Phone

Smiling on the phone means giving voice cues that tell clients you are happy to hear from them. Using pleasant tones, being extra courteous, and actively listening are a few suggestions to improve phone communication. Actually smiling when the phone rings is a great way to heighten your attitude before you speak to your caller.

Developing rapport on the phone will help you retain customers, and clients will be less likely to be upset when you need them to change appointments or wait for a technician who is running behind schedule.

Customer Service

Excellent customer service is imperative in the cosmetology business and probably more important when you are speaking to a client on the phone. The three C's of customer service (confidence, consideration, control) will guarantee the best customer service possible.

Be confident even when you don't have an answer. Simply tell the client you will find the answer and then do all you can to do so. Always express confidence when a client is upset. A displeased client needs to feel that the person she is talking to has some power to correct her problem. When you express confidence in all situations, clients on the other end of the line feel like they can count on you to get the job done. How much confidence would you have in the technician in the following dialogue?

Technician:	*Computerworld, this is Grant.*
Customer:	*Hello, Grant, I need to get a tape backup for my computer. Do you sell them?*
Technician:	*Yeah, I think we sell them.*
Customer:	*Can you tell me approximately how much it will cost?*
Technician:	*Well, I really don't know right off hand.*
Customer:	*Grant, can you tell me if your company installs them?*
Technician:	*Yeah, I know we do that.*
Customer:	*How long does that take? I use my computer daily in my business so I can't be without it for very long. Can someone come here to install the tape backup?*
Technician:	*Oh, no we don't do that. I think it takes at least three days.*
Customer:	*Thank you, Grant, I'll try another store.*

Would you purchase from Grant's store?

Be considerate of your clients' feelings. Realize that it is frustrating to clients when they can't get an appointment at the most convenient time for them. Try to see situations from your client's viewpoint. It's easy to get a little angry when your stylist is ill and you have to rearrange your schedule. It can be scary for clients to get their first perm, or to get their long hair cut short, or to commit to permanent color. Even a broken fingernail can be a disaster to a client if her nail tech can't repair it immediately. When you care about your customer, the attitude is carried through in your voice.

Always be in control. Project a positive image over the phone by speaking in a professional, enthusiastic voice. Learn everything about your company, its services, and its products so that you can answer every question or at least know where to go to get the answer. Keep updated and aware of changes in your salon, promotions, and specials you are offering and be creative when scheduling appointments—look for all the options to get what the client wants.

No matter how good you think you sound to your clients, it's the customer's perception that counts. It's what the customer hears that matters, not what we say. If a client says the receptionist was rude on the phone, apologize even if you know that your receptionist is the most caring person on your staff. When a client insists she was told that your skin care special ran through next week when it really ends this week, offer your regrets that a mistake was made and negotiate with her.

Clarifying communication is your responsibility, not the caller's. In the following conversation, look for ways you could be more clear than Margo.

Margo: *Good morning, Sensations Salon, this is Margo. How may I help you?*

Caller: *Hi, I would like to have an appointment to get my color done. Monique does it for me.*

Margo: *Monique has time Wednesday the 12th at 10 A.M.*

Caller: *I can't do that. I work at that time.*

Margo: *We have time on Thursday afternoon. Monique is open at four o'clock.*

Caller: *No, that isn't good either. That's just when my kids get home.*

Margo: *Well, how about Wednesday evening?. She has 7 P.M. available.*

Caller: *Yes, that's good. Wednesday at 7 P.M.*

Margo: *Now, wait a minute, that's next week not this week. OK, now what's your name?*

Caller: *This is Susan White.*

Margo: *I have you scheduled for Wednesday the 12th at 7 P.M. to get your hair colored, right? And that's all you need done?*

Caller: *No, I also need my hair cut.*

Margo: *Well, that changes things. Why didn't you tell me in the first*

> *No matter how good you think you sound to your clients, it's the customer's perception that counts.*

> *place? You'll have to come in at 6:45 P.M. then or she won't have enough time.*

Caller: *It usually takes her a long time to do my color. Are you sure she has enough time for it?*

Margo: *Do you have long hair or something?*

Caller: *No, it's shoulder length, but she weaves in three different colors.*

Margo: *Oh, you're talking about a foil weave color. That's a different story. She can't do that at all on Wednesday . . .*

Margo could have built better rapport by asking for Susan's name in the beginning of the conversation and using it as she scheduled the appointment. By finding out the type of color service Susan gets and whether she needed any other services, Margo would have used much less time to schedule Susan's appointment. Furthermore, if Margo had found out when Susan was available rather than suggesting many different times that didn't work for Susan, an appointment could have been scheduled without the frustration that both parties experienced.

Your Telephone Voice

A speaking rate of 100 to 120 words per minute is considered slow, while 130 to 150 words per minute is average and 180 to 200 is fast. Imagine listening to someone whose words tumble out at a very fast rate. Would you feel that the speaker was in a hurry? Consider someone who speaks so slowly that you become an impatient listener. When you are speaking on the phone to a client who speaks slowly, slow down your rate of speech to match your client. Speed up your rate to match a client who speaks quickly. The only time you should not mirror your client's speech rate is when he is angry or hysterical.

Don't speak with an irritated voice. No matter which words you select, an irritated voice communicates "What do you want now?" Even when a client calls back to change an appointment for the fourth time, don't sound agitated. Treat that client like he is the most important client you have talked to today.

When you speak on the phone, your voice loses about 30% of its energy simply because of transmission through phone lines. Your otherwise pleasant voice can sound flat and uncaring. Add extra positive energy to your voice and you will see a big difference in your caller's level of cooperation.

Don't be apathetic—it's contagious. If you're having difficulty keeping a great attitude, try taking a sixty-second vacation away from the phone. Take a break where you can be alone. Breathe deeply, relax, and realize that you don't have to be affected by other people's negativity.

Assertive or Aggressive Messages

Aggressive statements will often be intimidating to clients and act as barriers to building rapport. Assertive statements can say the same thing as aggressive statements; however, assertive statements say it without offense. To be assertive, use sharing words as opposed to the aggressive intimidating commentary. Assertive remarks use *I* statements, while aggressive ones use *you* statements.

Assertive statements can say the same thing as aggressive statements; however, assertive statements say it without offense.

Aggressive Statements

You'll have to wait. He is busy right now.

You can't do it that way. You have to get the perm first.

You'll have to get a clarifying treatment before your perm.

Assertive Statements

Please wait while I find out how long he will be.

We feel we get better results by cutting after the perm.

We do a clarifying treatment before the perm because . . .

Answering the Phone

How many times should the phone ring before you answer it? If you answer immediately on the first ring, you can startle callers. They might feel like you are sitting on the phone ready to pounce as soon as it begins to ring. Answering after two rings is ideal;

however, in a busy salon it's not as practical as answering on the third ring. When you answer on the fourth ring, clients are wondering where you are. If you answer after four rings, be sure to express a lot of positive energy to the client.

Amazingly, during the first ten seconds on the phone, clients decide if they like or dislike you and whether to trust you. That first impression happens before you even get a chance at customer service.

To assure that your salon gives a good impression, standardize the greeting procedure for all salon staff who answer the phone. "Good morning or afternoon" is nice to hear; however, if you are unaware of the time, it's easy to make a mistake. Simply state your company name and then your name. Avoid saying "Margo speaking." Obviously, you are speaking if the client is hearing you. Instead say, "This is Margo." Next, ask how you can be of service to the customer. For example, "Sensations Salon, this is Margo. How may I help you?"

Keep your salon greeting short and to the point. Did you ever listen to a greeting that was so involved you forgot what you called about? For example, "Good afternoon, you have reached Sensations Hair and Skin Care Salon and Day Spa. Salon of the year for 1995 and recognized by the World Colorist Association as a master color salon. How may I help you?"

Qualify the caller by listening for what the caller wants and the type of caller. Do they need information, require action, or are they in sales? Are they clients, prospective clients, or another type of caller? In an information call, the caller needs information about your salon, such as prices and the types of services or products you offer. An action call requires you to take some form of action. Scheduling an appointment, confirming an appointment, canceling an appointment, and special ordering a product for a client are all action calls. In a sales call, the caller is selling a product or service. Anyone who has spent any time at all as a receptionist is aware of the many sales calls that come through the switchboard daily. Thorough knowledge of which dealers your company uses will help you screen sales calls.

When you have determined that the call is client oriented, your next objective is to get the client's name. "May I ask who is calling?" is the simplest way of getting the client's name. If you have trouble remembering names, use the client's name right away or jot it down on a piece of scrap paper.

Answering the phone after two rings is ideal; however in a busy salon it's not as practical as answering on the third ring.

If your salon has multiple phone lines, there will be times when you have to put clients on hold. If you ask permission to put a client on hold, wait for the answer before you push the hold button. If you simply say "please hold," be careful to say it with a pleasant voice. Thirty to forty-five seconds is the maximum you should keep someone on hold before getting back to them. If the client must hold longer than sixty seconds, offer to call back if the client doesn't want to remain on hold.

In a situation where you are the only receptionist and you have a client to check out and schedule for his next appointment, a delivery that is C.O.D, and both incoming lines ringing, what is your priority?

The highest priority is to keep a calm, even voice. Don't allow anyone to think they are being rushed through (accept the delivery person). Then follow whatever procedure is outlined by your salon.

Callers are potential sales, and the objective of your business is to make sales. Never make waiting clients feel they are less important than the caller; however, the client on the phone can't see how busy you are. One way is to enroll the client in your dilemma by asking if the client you are checking out can wait just a minute while you take your calls.

Margo: *Could you wait just a minute while I take these calls?*

Client: *I'm really in a hurry right now.*

Margo: *OK. I'll just ask them to hold while I check you out.*

Client: *Sure.*

or

Margo: *Could you wait just a minute while I take these calls?*

Client: *Sure, go ahead.*

Margo: *Good morning, Sensations Salon. This is Margo. How can I help you?*

Caller 1: *This is Donna Appleby. I need an appointment with Carl.*

Margo: *Hi, Donna. Hold just a minute please. I'll be right back.*

Margo: *Good morning, Sensations Salon. This is Margo. How can I help you?*

Caller 2: *I'd like to get a haircut with Janet.*

Margo: *Sure, who is calling please?*

Caller 2: *This is James White.*

Margo: *Please hold, James, I'm scheduling on another line. I'll be right back.*

Caller 2. *OK.*

Scheduling Appointments

A script for scheduling appointments is probably the most valuable script you will utilize in your salon. To save time on the phone, create an appointment script made up of closed questions, giving the client options requiring short responses, a yes or no answer, or specific choices.

Outline the information you require to schedule an appointment. You will need the client's name, the services required, whether a stylist is requested, when the client and the preferred stylist are available, and the client's phone number.

A simple scheduling script can be attached to the reception desk in such a way that it is seen every time someone answers the phone. Here is a sample scheduling script (the client's responses have been omitted):

Receptionist: *Sensations Salon, this is (name of receptionist). How may I help you?*
May I ask who is calling?

(Client's name), have you been to our salon before?
What services do you need?
Is there a stylist you would prefer?
(Client's name), when are you available?
(Find an agreeable appointment time.)
May I have a phone number where we can confirm
your appointment the day before?
(Confirm services, day, date, time, and the stylist or technician.)
Thank you, (client's name). Good bye.

Here is an example of a scheduling script in action:

Customer: *I need an appointment for a haircut.*

Receptionist: *May I ask who is calling, please?*

Customer: *Yes, this is Jackie Johnson.*

Receptionist: *Is there a particular stylist you would like to cut your hair?*

Customer: *Monique usually cuts my hair, but John does OK too.*

Receptionist: *Jackie, are you available during the day or do you need an evening appointment?*

Customer: *I'm only available between twelve thirty and three thirty. Can I have an appointment this week?*

Receptionist: *John has an opening on Friday at one o'clock or Monique has a two o'clock on Thursday. Would either appointment be convenient?*

Customer: *Yes, that is great. I'll take the one o'clock with John.*

Receptionist: *Jackie, may I have a phone number where I can reach you the day before your appointment?*

Customer: *Just leave a message on my recorder. The number is . . .*

Receptionist: *OK, Jackie, you are scheduled for a haircut with John at two o'clock on Friday the sixth. That's this Friday.*

Customer: *Great. See you then.*

A script for sheduling appointments is probably the most valuable script you will utilize in your salon.

The previous dialogue changes dramatically when a receptionist combines a selling script with the appointment script.

Receptionist: *Would either appointment be convenient?*

Customer: *Yes, that is great. I'll take the one o'clock with John.*

Receptionist: *Jackie, this month we have a special promotion for our preferred clients. You can get a mini-scalp massage free when you get a moisturizing treatment. Doesn't that sound wonderful? It's only fifteen dollars. It takes about fifteen or twenty minutes, so we would have to have you come in a little earlier. Can you come in at 1:45 on Friday?*

Customer: *Yes, I can make it. My hair does seem a little dry in this winter weather.*

Before receptionists can sell additional services, they must have a written script in front of them with a list of features and benefits so they can maintain control of the conversation.

Do clients ever say no to your script? Of course they do. And don't be surprised if some days you have more no responses than yes responses.

Pricing Inquiry Calls

If your caller merely wants information, it is as important to give value and service information about your salon as it is to quote salon prices. Always quote the maximum price for the service or give the inquirer a price range. If your answer to an inquiry is "A haircut is forty-five dollars," the prospective client doesn't have a clue about the difference between your forty-five-dollar haircut and a twenty-five-dollar haircut down the street.

Margo: *Good morning, Sensations Salon, Margo speaking. May I help you?*

Caller: *Hello, could you please tell me the price of a perm?*

Margo: *Of course, I can do that! Who am I speaking to?*

Caller: *This is Pamela. I've never been to your salon. I just want to know the price of a perm.*

Margo: *Hi, Pamela. I can give you a price range for a perm. It will be between seventy-five and ninety-five dollars depending on the length and texture of your hair. You see, here at Sensations Salon, we want to be sure that your hair is thoroughly analyzed before we perm it. And since everyone's hair has different requirements and we want to be sure your perm here is the best you have ever had, we can't give you an exact price over the phone. I can tell you, however, that all perms include hair and scalp analysis and an intensive treatment according to what your hair needs. Consultations at our salon are free. Could you come in today or tomorrow for free consultation or would you rather schedule now for the perm and consultation?*

Caller: *Sure, I could do that. I work during the day, however. Can I have something in the evening for the consultation?*

or

Caller: *I'd really rather not schedule anything yet.*

Margo: *If you could give me your address, I would gladly mail you a complete salon brochure. That way you can see all the different services we offer.*

If your caller merely wants information, it is as important to give value and service information about your salon as it is to quote salon prices.

Confirmation Calls

Confirmation calls remind clients of upcoming appointments and give the salon an opportunity to add services to the next day's schedule. Many progressive salons are using confirmation calls the day before to remind clients of appointments. Confirming also reinforces the professionalism of the salon and avoids last-minute cancellations of those people who forgot or weren't going to call and cancel until the last minute.

Margo: *This is Margo from Sensations Salon calling to confirm (or remind you about) your appointment for a color and haircut tomorrow with Marc at 2:45.*

Cathy: *Yes, Margo, I have it on my calendar. I'll be there.*

Margo: *Cathy, would you like to have a manicure while your color is processing? We have an extraordinary new treatment for exfoliating and moisturizing your hands, and I know you'll love it. Your hands will feel like baby skin for days. Would you like to try it?*

Cathy: *How much does it cost?*

Margo: *The manicure is twelve and the hand treatment is an additional five.*

Cathy: *Sure. I'll try it. I have to sit there while the color works anyway, so I might as well be pampered.*

Margo: *Great, Cathy. I know you'll love it!*

Follow-Up Calls

Follow-up calls can be made to clients who have made significant style, color, or perm changes, to clients who get a new service, and to clients who are due for services. To most people, sales calls from telemarketing companies are bothersome and become irritating, especially at mealtimes. However, because of the intimacy of the relationship between salon professionals and clients, the sound of a stylist's voice on the phone can conjure up good feelings.

A few days after their appointment, call clients to be sure that they are happy with their new color, perm, or other service. Follow-up calls strengthen your relationship with clients by giving them the message that you care about the results of your work.

Suzanne: *Hello, Roxie, this is Suzanne from Sensations Salon. I was just calling to find out how you liked the AHA treatment I gave you Saturday.*

Roxie: *Oh, Suzanne. That was everything you said it would be. My skin looks wonderful. I can't wait to get my next facial.*

Suzanne: *I'm glad you liked it, Roxie. Did you know that we have an AHA special package? You get the series of six mini-*

facial treatments for 200 dollars. I think you would enjoy them.

Roxie: *You told me about it when you gave me the facial. I'd love to do it, but I just don't have time to get in there every week.*

Suzanne: *How about during your lunch break? You work just a few minutes from here and we could get your treatments done in thirty minutes.*

Roxie: *Are you sure I can get done in thirty minutes. What if you are running behind schedule or something?*

Suzanne: *I will schedule you so that I won't be running late and if something unforeseen happens, I'll have Margo call you.*

Roxie: *Sounds good, and if I bring my lunch I'll still have time for a quick bite before I go back to work. But what about my makeup? I can't go back to work without my makeup on.*

A few days after their appointment, call clients to be sure that they are happy with their new color, perm, or other service.

Suzanne: *We can do a quick makeup on you. It will take about ten minutes.*

Roxie: *That really makes a tight schedule. Maybe I'll bring my makeup and do it when I get back to work.*

Suzanne: *That sounds like it will work. Let's get this scheduled for you. How about the same day every week? How are Tuesdays?*

Roxie: *Tuesday sounds great.*

Clients who fail to schedule in advance often wait too long before calling for their appointment. Sometimes they wait so long that we are sure we have lost them. Then they call, needing an appointment right away because they are severely overdue. Follow-up calls can get them into the salon on schedule. Check back four or five weeks ago in your appointment book to find those clients that will be due for a service. If your salon is computerized, you can get that same list with just the push of a few buttons.

Marc: *Hello, may I speak to Jack Young please?*

Jack: *Speaking.*

Marc: *This is Marc Hammond from Sensations Salon. How are you today?*

Jack: *Busy. What can I do for you?*

Marc: *Jack, it has been four weeks since your last haircut and your hair is probably getting long. I'm calling to see if you would like to schedule for a haircut before your hair gets too out of hand.*

Jack: *You're right, it is long. Do you have time tomorrow after 5:00?*

Marc: *How about 5:30?*

Jack: *Sounds great. Thanks, Marc.*

What happens if the client doesn't want to schedule an appointment?

Marc: *Jack, it has been four weeks since your last haircut and your hair is probably getting long. I'm calling to see if you would like to schedule for a haircut before your hair gets too out of hand.*

Jack: *Actually, Marc, I'm kind of enjoying it with more length. I think I'll let it grow a few more weeks.*

Marc: *Sounds good, Jack. Even if you want more length in your style, you will still need a reshaping if you want to keep from looking unruly. How about if I ask our receptionist, Margo, to give you a call in, say, three weeks?*

Jack: *That will be fine, Marc. That way I don't have to think about it.*

Now Marc must be certain that either he or Margo calls in three weeks to schedule Jack's appointment.

There are many salon calls that we would rather not have to make. Scripting those calls makes the task easier and less stressful.

What do you say when an otherwise dependable client misses an appointment? Don't assume that it was the client's fault. After all, you don't know if the appointment was scheduled improperly or if she just forgot. By giving her the chance to take responsibility, you get an opportunity to get her back in the salon.

Margo: *Hello, Molly? This is Margo calling from Sensations Salon. We had you scheduled for a color and cut at ten this morning. Did we schedule you for the wrong day?*

When an otherwise dependable client misses an appointment, don't assume that it was the client's fault.

Accusing the client puts her on the defensive and can alienate her.

Margo: *Hello, Molly. You missed your appointment today.*

Molly: *Margo, I didn't have an appointment today. Can't you people get your appointments straight? I would never have scheduled for this morning. I work on Thursday mornings. My appointment is for Tuesday morning and it better be on your book. You know you're not the only salon in town!*

Notice the difference when you take responsibility for the mistake.

Margo: *Hello, Molly? This is Margo calling from Sensations Salon. We had you scheduled for a color and cut at ten this morning. Did we schedule it for the wrong day?*

Molly: *Hi, Margo. I didn't have an appointment today. According to my calendar, it's Tuesday at ten. Can you make sure that is when I'm scheduled?*

Margo: *Oh Molly, I'm glad I called you. We really made a mistake on this one. We don't have you scheduled and Carl is already booked at that time. Is it possible for you to come at eleven on Tuesday instead of ten? I apologize for this.*

Molly: *That's OK, Margo, we all make mistakes.*

Calling to Reschedule

How do you deal with clients when their stylist is late or, worse, sick and you have to reschedule the entire day? First, don't use weak language. Rather than say "I'm sorry," say "I regret that has happened" or "I apologize."

Margo: *Hello, Mrs. Thomas. I'm calling to tell you that Marc will be a little late getting to you today. I just want to let you know and make sure that you allow an extra half hour in your schedule today.*

Margo: *Hello, Mrs. Thomas. I regret to tell you that we must reschedule your appointment because your stylist Marc is ill today. However, we have a few options. You can have an appointment with Patrick at the same time as you were scheduled with Marc, or we have a few openings with other staff members later in the day. Or, if you wish, we can reschedule you with Marc for another day.*

Above all, do not let the client off the phone without scheduling another appointment. Should the worst occur and you don't get another appointment scheduled, be sure to jot down the client's name and phone number so the stylist can get back to her.

What Do You Say When a Client Cancels?

No matter how good we are at scheduling and confirming appointments, there will always be some unavoidable cancellations. The goal in a cancellation call is to get the appointment back in the book as soon as possible.

Marilyn: *Hello, Margo, this is Marilyn, I have an appointment with Monique at four and I can't make it. I have a meeting at school that I wasn't aware of. I'm sorry about that.*

Margo: *Hi, Marilyn. I'm sorry you can't get here today. How about scheduling for Friday? Wendy had a cancellation at four-thirty.*

Marilyn: *I can't. I don't have my calendar.*

Margo: *I know it's difficult when you don't know your schedule; however, I know how you hate it when your hair is too long. You know it can be hard to get an appointment with Monique, so don't want to wait too long to call.*

Marilyn: *Well, maybe you should go ahead and give me that Friday appointment. I'll rearrange things if I have to.*

A simple reminder that the caller might not be able to get the time she wants can be an incentive to make her hair appointment a priority.

The goal in a cancellation call is to get the appointment back in the book as soon as possible.

Salon Loyalty

Be loyal to your company. Don't blame anyone for mistakes: not staff members, not manufacturers of your products, and not the management. In some situations, company loyalty will require you to take responsibility yourself, even if a problem isn't yours.

Margo: *Good morning, Sensations Salon, this is Margo. How can I help you?*

Trisha: *Hello, Margo. I have an appointment for my highlight and cut at eleven tomorrow. You weren't there when I scheduled it last week. The person I spoke to said I would be out of there by 12:30. I have a very important meeting to go to, so I want to look really good. After I thought about it, I realized that it always takes more than an hour and a half to do my color and cut. Can you check on it for me?*

Margo: *Let's see. You must be Trisha. You're scheduled with Carl for your highlight and Monique for your cut. You're right, though, you won't be finished by 12:30.*

Trisha: *Can I come earlier, then?*

Margo: *Carl is completely full all morning, and Monique doesn't have any flexible time either. Can we reschedule?*

Trisha: *No! I need to be done tomorrow. My hair looks awful and I have a very important meeting.*

At this point, Margo is wondering which staff member took this appointment, and who could have been so inept as to schedule it this way. She could blame this dilemma on the staff member who scheduled it. However, Margo is loyal to her company and chooses to take responsibility.

Margo: *I apologize for this mistake, Trisha. Let me see what I can do about it. Hold on just a minute, please.*

Margo (returning to the phone): *Trisha, I checked with Carl. He is willing to come in at 8:00 A.M. tomorrow to get your highlighting done. However, I still can't get you into Monique's schedule. Marc has an opening for a cut after your highlight, if you would like to switch to him.*

In some situations, company loyalty will require you to take responsibility for yourself, even if a problem isn't yours.

Trisha: *Monique has a plan for my hair, so I don't want to switch stylists, but how about if I don't get cut tomorrow and just get styled after my color?*

Margo: *That will work great for us, Trisha. See you tomorrow at 8 o'clock in the morning.*

In another situation, Margo is on the phone with a customer complaining that her son's haircut isn't right.

Mrs. Grovener: *Hello, Margo? This is Mrs. Grovener. My Robbie came home from your salon in tears yesterday. His haircut isn't what he asked for. It's much too short on top and not nearly short enough on the sides and in the back. That new girl, Jennifer, I think her name was, cut it. She sure did a lousy job.*

Margo: *I regret that that happened to Robbie, Mrs. Grovener. It's upsetting to see your child unhappy. This is an unusual occurrence for Jennifer. She typically spends a lot of time consulting. I apologize for the lack of communication. What can I do to help?*

Mrs. Grovener: *It has to be fixed right away. Can Marc do it? He always does such a great job with my hair.*

Margo: *Ordinarily, we would like Jennifer to see what's wrong with her haircut, but she isn't here today. It looks like Marc can work you into his schedule today right after school, at about 4:15. How's that?*

Mrs. Grovener: *Great, Margo, that will work. Thanks!*

Margo: *Thanks for calling, Mrs. Grovener. I'm glad we could take care of Robbie.*

In a situation like this, avoid statements like the following:

"He's new, and you know how it is when you're just starting out?"

"It isn't the first time this has happened."

"You say she did a lousy haircut . . ."

"She should have known better."

"I wouldn't trust him either."

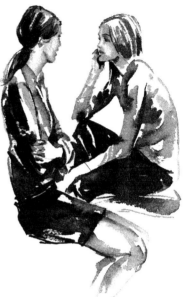

Another salon situation in which it's important for the person answering the phone to accept responsibility is in scheduling appointments.

Caller: *Hello, this is JoAnne Wilkes. May I speak to the manager, please?*

Margo: *Hello, JoAnne, this is Margo. Our manager is out of the salon today. Perhaps I can help you.*

Caller: *Margo, I came to your salon last night for my regular two-week fills and I had to wait thirty minutes for my appointment. I don't mind waiting every once in a while, but lately I have had to wait twenty to thirty minutes every time. Carolyn does a great job on my nails, but I feel like I have been taken advantage of and I've decided to go to another salon. Cancel my next appointment.*

What could the receptionist say? She could avoid any involvement and blame everyone else for the problem:

"The evening receptionist messed up the appointment ahead of yours . . ."

"Carolyn has been squeezing in too many people lately. I told her it was going to cause trouble . . ."

"I don't blame you, JoAnne. I'd switch to another nail tech, too."

Or she can be loyal to her co-workers and salon, knowing that every client is valuable and she should do whatever it takes to keep that client.

Margo: *I apologize for your inconvenience, JoAnne. We like to have our staff run on schedule, and since you have been a client for quite a while, you know that it is unusual for any client to wait more than a few minutes.*

JoAnn: *A few minutes I can handle, but half an hour is ridiculous. I'm not going to do it again.*

Margo: *Perhaps we need to find out what has happened. Carolyn is a marvelous nail tech, and she would be very disturbed if you stopped coming to her. Let me find out why you've had to wait so long. I'm sure there is a solution to this situation. Can I talk to Carolyn and get back to you? She gets in at twelve today, so I'll call you before two o'clock.*

JoAnn: *All right, Margo. Go ahead and talk to her, but I'll call you back at two. I'm not sure where I'll be at that time.*

Margo: *JoAnne, thanks for bringing this to our attention. I'll talk to you at two. Good-bye.*

Indecisive Clients

Did you ever have to deal with people who didn't know what they want? It's easy to sound impatient when clients don't know what services they want or what day or time is good for an appointment. These are the times when you feel like hanging up on the client.

The secret to handling indecisive clients is to ask closed questions instead of giving the client choices. When you say to an indecisive client, "When would you like to have your appointment?" he will reply, "Well, I don't know. When is your salon open?"

When you say, "Would you like to have Wednesday at 8:00 P.M., Thursday at 10:00 A.M., or Friday at noon?" the indecisive client won't be able to make up his mind. Instead ask him, "Are you available during the day?" If he says yes, continue with "Would you like to schedule for Thursday at 10:00 A.M.?" Pursue with closed questions until the appointment is scheduled and reconfirmed.

Also consider the client who doesn't want to stop talking. How do you interrupt or end a conversation without offending the client? Sometimes you have to interrupt; however, apologize for it and go on with business. Ask her a question that brings the conversation back to business. Stay in control of the conversation and use the client's name to interrupt when the client is talking too much or for too long. Close the conversation by reconfirming the appointment schedule.

Barb:	*How are you, Margo? This is Barb. I just called to get an appointment with Monique to have my hair shampooed and styled for the Silver Ball. It's on Saturday the 22nd. Anytime before two is a good time for me. I'd also like Suzanne to do my makeup and Carolyn to give me a manicure. I don't think I'll need a haircut yet, but maybe a little trim around the front. Hasn't this weather been just awful? I was out earlier today and . . .*
Margo:	*Barb, excuse me for interrupting. How would you like to have a ten o'clock appointment? It looks like we can fit in everything you need. How does that sound?*
Barb:	*Great, ten o'clock is just perfect. I sure hope I get over this cold by then. I've been dragging it around for a week. Do I still sound hoarse to you? My throat is much better than it was yesterday . . .*
Margo:	*Excuse me again, Barb. I just want to be sure I have this scheduled properly. You need a style with Monique, makeup with Suzanne, and a manicure with Carolyn. We have that all on Saturday the 22nd at ten o'clock. Am I correct?*
Barb:	*Yes, that's right, Margo.*
Margo:	*Great. I hope your cold is better by then. Thanks for calling Barb. Good-bye.*

The secret to handling indecisive clients is to ask closed questions instead of giving the client choices.

Screening Calls and Messages

The majority of calls into the salon are from clients needing appointments. However, there are other types of calls, such as personal calls for staff members, sales calls, and calls from charitable organizations that also require scripting to be handled quickly and efficiently.

Taking Messages

When you are in a busy salon with multiple phone lines, it's important to get all the information for a message as quickly as possible. A message pad is helpful for this. Ask closed questions when possible. Find out the first and last name and the complete phone number. Even if the caller says, "This is George and she knows my number," get the full name and number anyway. Jot down the time of the call and ask the nature of the message. It's also a good idea to find out when the staff member can call back.

Sometimes you get persistent callers who insist on speaking to their stylist. If it is salon policy that stylists not be interrupted when servicing a client, you must find a tactful way to satisfy the persistent caller. The following dialogue will help you deal with this situation.

Receptionist:	*I'm sorry, Carl isn't available right now. May I take a message? Or, Carl is working with a client right now and can't break away. May I take a message?*
Persistent caller:	*I have to talk to him right now.*
Receptionist:	*May I ask who is calling? I can take a message to him and find out when he can get back to you.*
Persistent caller:	*Just go get him, I have to talk to him now.*

Receptionist:	*Are you a client of Carl's?*
Persistent caller:	*No, this is Mary Ann, his cousin.*
Receptionist:	*Oh, hello, Mary Ann, is this a family emergency?*
Persistent caller:	*No. It's not an emergency, I just have to talk to him now.*
Receptionist:	*Mary Ann, Carl is applying haircolor and it's difficult to leave a client at that stage. There are two things I can do. I can give him your message and call you back in just a few minutes to tell you what he said, or I can look at his schedule and tell you when he will have a break so you can call him back.*
Persistent caller:	*I'm not in a place where you can call me, so I guess you'll have to tell me when I can call him.*

When you are in a busy salon with multiple phone lines, it's important to get all the information for a message as quickly as possible.

Another caller who can be difficult is the persistent sales caller.

Margo:	*Sensations Salon, this is Margo. May I help you?*
Caller:	*Yes, Margo. I'd like to speak to the manager.*
Margo:	*Yes, how may I help you?*
Caller:	*Are you the manager?*
Margo:	*I have many responsibilities in the salon. Please tell me the nature of your call and I will either help you or direct your call to the right person.*
Caller:	*I need to speak to the person who purchases your janitorial supplies.*
Margo:	*Yes, I can probably help you with that. May I ask who is calling and what company you are with?*

Part of Margo's responsibility is to screen calls. When the manager or owner of your salon is also a key staff member serving clients, sales calls must be screened and directed to another staff member who can help.

Message Call Backs

Did you ever wait by a phone for someone who said they would call back ASAP and an hour later you were angrily still waiting? The expression ASAP means as soon as possible, and the term is relative. To one person it could mean five minutes, to someone else it could mean tomorrow or the next day. Instead of saying ASAP, use a specific time. For example, "I will call you back before ten tomorrow or before the end of the business day." Then be sure to call back, even if it is only to let the person know that you don't have the information she wanted yet.

Not returning calls is rude and discourteous. Always return messages, even if you have to have someone else do it for you. In addition, avoid telephone tag by finding out the availability of the other person and by stating a time when you will be available.

Displeased Clients

Clients will express things over the phone that they would never say face to face. For some reason, they are braver speaking over the phone, so most complaints will come in the form of a phone call. When an angry or upset client calls, deal with the anger immediately using these rules:

1. Don't buy into it. The worst situation is for you to get angry also. Consider the source and realize that some people have been angry since birth.

2. Listen, even when you don't agree with what the client is saying. To help justify their anger, angry people will sometimes exaggerate a situation. Try to listen without judging.

3. Show empathy for the client's feelings. Acknowledge the client's emotions and repeat the content of the client's complaint. Several things happen when you give feedback to an angry client. Simply knowing that she has been heard will calm her, and your client's complaint restated in your neutral voice can make the situation look different.

4. Identify what the client needs and wants. Don't offer to give the client anything; instead ask her what she would like you to do. Often, a client doesn't ask for nearly as much as you would give her.

5. Offer options. Tell the client all the ways that you could help her with her problem.

6. Move to a positive solution. Agree on the best course of action, and make arrangements for the solution to happen.

7. Always thank the client for calling and giving you the opportunity to take care of the problem.

8. Always follow up to be sure the client is satisfied.

A client calls the salon and says in a loud, angry voice, "Hello, I'm Edna. Campbell. This perm Carl gave me last week just isn't right. My last perm was soft, just like natural wave. This one is dry and horrible. What did he do to me?"

Receptionist Margo: *I'm sorry that you're not happy with your perm, Mrs. Campbell.*

Mrs. Campbell: *You bet I'm not happy. What are you going to do about it?*

Margo: *Mrs. Campbell, if your hair is dry because of a perm that we did, then I understand your disappointment. We will do whatever it takes to get your hair back in good shape. When are you available to get started? We would like to analyze your hair so we know what treatment it will need.*

Mrs. Campbell: *I want something done right away if you have time.*

Margo: *Carl could consult with you at three this afternoon. Can you make that?*

Mrs. Campbell: *That's good. Thanks, Margo, I'll be there.*

Margo: *Thank you for calling, Mrs. Campbell. I'll see you this afternoon.*

Two days later, Margo or Carl make a check up call on Mrs. Campbell. For example, "Hi, Mrs. Campbell. This is Carl from Sensations Salon. I'm calling to see how your hair is doing now."

Debbie Raffill

Salon 2000

Madison, WI

In our salon, when a client calls or stops in because they aren't happy with their service, the desk coordinators write out a grievance form and turn the client over to a manager. If the problem is simply a minor adjustment in a cut, we schedule for a recut without the manager's intervention. However, we still fill out a grievance form so we can track displeased clients. It's a good idea to check back to be sure the client is satisfied with the redo.

When displeased clients' problems are corrected to their satisfaction and clients feel that you really care that they are satisfied, you will gain a more loyal client than ever before.

Chapter Summary

1. Smiling on the phone means giving voice cues that tell clients you are happy to hear from them. Using pleasant tones, being extra-courteous, and actively listening are a few suggestions to improve phone communication. Actually smiling when the phone rings is a great way to heighten your attitude before you speak to your caller.

2. The three C's of customer service that guarantee the best customer service are confidence, consideration, and control.

3. No matter how good you think you sound to your clients, it's the customer's perception that counts. It's what the customer hears that matters, not what we say.

4. When you are speaking on the phone to a client who speaks slowly, slow down your rate of speech to match your client. Speed up your rate to match a client who speaks quickly. The only time you should not mirror your client's speech rate is when he is angry or hysterical.

5. During the first ten seconds on the phone, clients decide if they like or dislike you and whether to trust you. That first impression happens before you even get a chance at customer service.

6. A script for scheduling appointments is probably the most valuable script you will utilize in your salon. To save time on the phone, create an appointment script made up of closed questions, giving the client options requiring short responses, a yes or no answer, or specific choices.

7. If you have identified a caller as one who merely wants information, it is as important to give value and service information about your salon as it is to quote salon prices.

8. Confirmation calls remind clients of upcoming appointments and give the salon an opportunity to add services to the next day's schedule.

9. There are many salon calls that we would rather not have to make. Scripting calls, such as to clients who have missed appointments, makes the task easier and less stressful.

10. No matter how good we are at scheduling and confirming appointments, there will always be some unavoidable cancellations. The goal in a cancellation call is to get the appointment back in the book as soon as possible.

Reception

Scheduling Appointments

Margo: *Maggie, you look great. I really like that new haircolor. What can I do for you?*

Maggie: *I just dropped by to pick up some hairspray and schedule some appointments.*

Margo: *You are already scheduled for your next cut, aren't you?*

Maggie: *Yes, I am. I want to schedule a facial and pedicure for my daughter and me. It's a gift for her. She's going to have a baby.*

Margo: *That's your first grandchild, isn't it? You must be really excited. When is it due?*

Maggie: *Oh, not until November. They find out so early these days, don't they?*

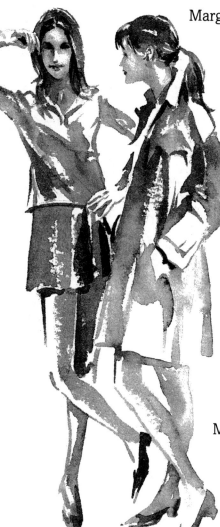

Margo: *Yes, they do. You want to get a pedicure and a manicure?*

Maggie: *No, I want a facial and a pedicure.*

Margo: *OK. When do you want it?*

Maggie: *On her birthday, June 15th.*

Margo: *We can do you both at 10 A.M. Would you like to have your makeup done after the facial?*

Maggie: *That sounds good. Do you think we'll be finished by 1:00 P.M.?*

Margo: *Yes. You'll be finished at about one. Are you taking her to lunch?*

Maggie: *Yes, we are going to spend the whole day together.*

Margo: *Here is an appointment card for you. It's at ten o'clock in the morning on June 15th.*

Maggie: *Thanks, Margo.*

Salons have general rules about scheduling, such as a half hour for a cut and an hour and a half for a perm. However, society has become so used to customization that we must also customize the way we schedule appointments. In the days when every hairstyle was a copy of the previous one, salons could schedule everyone the same way. Now, all our clients are different, and we perform several types of perming services and a multitude of coloring services. A client can choose a variety of nail services and even different polishing methods, such as regular polish or a French manicure.

When a client calls your salon to get her hair colored, you might think she means single-process color, just to cover the gray. However, what happens if she is thinking highlighting and her hair is 24 inches long? She appears at your salon near the end of a very busy Saturday—the same Saturday you plan to leave early for your cousin's wedding reception. Do you blame the client for not using the correct words when she scheduled her appointment? No. The fault really lies in the scheduling. Even on the busiest of days, it is important to ask all the questions that you need to get all the information as quickly as possible.

Suzanne: *Good morning, Sensations Salon. This is Suzanne. How may I help you?*

Barbara: *This is Barbara Collins. Isn't Margo there today?*

Suzanne: *Yes, she's here. I'm just filling in for her while she takes a short break. What can I do for you?*

Barbara (her voice is hurried and her words are curt): *I need to get an appointment for my color, cut, and nails. That would be with Carl, Monique, and Carolyn respectively. I must have it on Saturday the 29th of May between ten and two.*

Suzanne: *OK, let me get the book to the 29th. Here we are. Oh, this looks good. We can start you at 10:15 with Carl for your color, then you will get your nails done, and finally your cut with Monique. How does that sound?*

Barbara: *Sounds perfect. Saturday, the 29th at 10:15. Good-bye.*

Margo: *Thank you for taking over for me, Suzanne. I'm sorry I took so long. Anything happen while I was gone?*

Suzanne: *Not really. Just regular calls. Barbara Collins just called. She certainly has a controlling personality, doesn't she? She knows exactly what she wants and when she wants it. Fortunately, there was time open when she wanted it. I would hate to tell her she can't get an appointment when she wants it.*

Margo: *You're right, Suzanne. She can be difficult. Where did you schedule her?*

Suzanne: *Here, on May 29th.*

Margo: *Uh, oh. Barbara wears sculptured nails. That takes more time than the manicure you scheduled for her. She also gets lowlighting after her root color. I'll have to call her to rearrange the schedule. Oh—you forgot to get her phone number. That's OK, I'll get it from the computer.*

Salons have general rules about scheduling, such as a half hour for a cut and an hour and a half for a perm. However, society has become so used to customization that we must also customize the way we schedule appointments.

Suzanne: Wow, I'm sorry, Margo. I really messed up that one. I know we always get phone numbers, but she was just so demanding, she threw me off balance.

Margo: She can't bite you through the phone lines, Suzanne. Remember next time always to ask what kind of color they get and what kind of nail service. If you are scheduling a perm, always find out how long the hair is. It takes more time to do long hair. OK?

Suzanne: I guess if I was a stylist instead of an esthetician, I would know all that.

Margo: No, Suzanne. Even the stylists don't think to ask all the right questions.

The Receptionist's Relationship with Salon Personnel

To complicate matters for a receptionist, salon personnel work at different rates. Inexperienced personnel usually require additional time for services, while accomplished personnel all work at different speeds. It is easy to say that your salon has a scheduling policy of specific time allowances for each service. However, an alert receptionist will be aware of those staff members who need extra time here and there to catch up and those staff members who can work in an extra client.

The receptionist also works closely with both the salon staff and the clients and must often choose between making a client happy and inconveniencing staff members.

Suzanne's client, Victoria, is scheduled for a facial at 11:30. She is calling Margo to tell her that she will be late.

An alert receptionist will be aware of those staff members who need extra time here and there to catch up and those staff members who can work in an extra client.

Victoria: Margo, I just got out of a meeting. Is it too late to come in for my facial? It will take me fifteen minutes to get there.

Margo: Looks like it will be all right. Suzanne has a lunch break after you, so she won't be running behind schedule.

Victoria: Thanks, Margo, I'll be right there.

Margo   (pages Suzanne):   Suzanne, your next client will be about twenty minutes late.

Suzanne: *Twenty minutes . . . and you told her that was all right? I had plans to go out for lunch.*

Margo: *Oh, I'm sorry, Suzanne. I guess I should have asked first. I just assumed that you wouldn't mind. You have lots of time for lunch later.*

Suzanne: *I do mind. Next time please ask.*

Since the entire salon business revolves around the salon appointment book, the person who controls the book also controls the business. It's a powerful position to be in and also a stressful one. Clients sometimes make almost impossible requests and salon personnel, with all their different work habits, make their various demands on the salon receptionist. To promote goodwill and teamwork, the salon receptionist needs to keep staff happy. To retain clients, the receptionist must make them happy. The two should work together well; however, that doesn't always occur.

Some common client demands are as follows:

Can't he work me in somehow?

When my (husband, children, secretary) calls, please give him (or her or them) this message.

I really like John, but I'd like to switch to Marc. How can I do that?

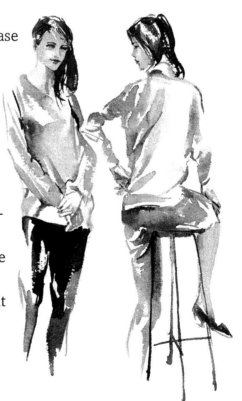

I have to get out of here in forty-five minutes. Would you get my stylist for me?

Can I postdate this check today?

Some common salon personnel demands are as follows:

Don't give me a lunch break; I need to take all the clients I can get this week.

Call Mrs. Smith and move her up. I don't want to wait around here all day just for her.

Don't book me. I want to leave early.

Go ahead and schedule me later.

You booked me too tight!

Where are all my clients?

Of course, the receptionist must always take care of those demands according to salon policy. However, it is important that the solution doesn't sever good working relationships.

Jennifer: *Margo, don't book me any more appointments, I want to leave early today.*

Margo: *Did you talk to Diane about it? I'll need her approval first.*

Jennifer: *Yeah, I'm going to check with her. I just wanted to make sure you knew so I don't get anymore clients today.*

Margo: *OK. Be sure to check with her right away.*

Jennifer: *Just as soon as I can.*

Minutes later, a desperate client calls, needing a perm and cut with anyone in the salon who can take her. Margo must decide how to keep everyone on good terms.

Margo puts the caller on hold and pages Jennifer.

Margo (to Jennifer): *I have a client who needs a perm and cut today. She can be here in ten minutes. I haven't heard from Diane about you leaving yet, so I have to give you this client. OK?*

Jennifer: *I just talked to Diane and she said it was OK to leave.*

Margo: *Jennifer, you are scheduled to work until five and I have a client that I have to give to you, and you know Diane would tell me to go ahead and book it. Sorry, but you'll have to stay.*

Jennifer: *I guess you're right.*

Sometimes the opposite happens.

Marc: *Margo, go ahead and start scheduling me later on Tuesdays and Thursdays. I'll take clients until 9:00 P.M.*

Margo: *That means you'll be working thirteen hours, three days in a row! I think you should talk to Diane about this.*

Marc: *It's my choice if I want to work more. Why should I have to ask her?*

Margo:	Because she's the salon manager, and I know she won't like it.
Marc:	This isn't going to be permanent. I need to bring in some extra money right now.
Margo:	I understand, but Diane schedules all staff members' work hours, so you have to go through her. OK?
Marc:	She is going to say no. She thinks I'll get burned out working so many hours. She gets upset if I even work through my lunch break.
Margo:	I have an idea, Marc. I think she will let you do it if you take extra breaks during the day—say, every five hours you take a half-hour break.
Marc:	That would defeat my purpose!
Margo:	You could still bring in more than in an eight-hour day. Besides, I think that's the only way she'll let you do it.
Marc:	You're probably right, Margo.

When a staff member says, "You booked me too tight! I can't work like that. I know I'll be running behind schedule all day!" a receptionist can respond, "I realize your schedule is a little tight today. How about if I speak to an assistant to be sure you get all the help you need?"

Sometimes staff members seem to accuse the receptionist of conspiring against them, as if it is solely the receptionist's job to get clients back into the salon.

Carolyn	(to Margo): Look at this schedule today. Why didn't you book me?
Margo:	It doesn't look like a busy day, does it?
Carolyn:	What happened to all my clients?
Margo:	If you would like to do something about those empty spaces, I can show you what to do.
Carolyn:	What?
Margo:	I can give a computer list of clients who are due for nail services if you would like to call them. It's a great way to get your schedule full!

When a Stylist Leaves the Salon

It's always an awkward situation when a staff member leaves the salon to go to another. At Sensations Salon, the policy is to tell inquiring clients where the staff member is now working. When handled with appropriate dialogue, the client is told the location and phone number of the staff member's new place of business. In addition, clients are given an incentive to stay with Sensations Salon.

The highest priority when a staff member leaves is to call all the clients who are already scheduled with that stay member.

Margo: *Good morning. May I speak to Jack Harley, please?*

Jack: *Speaking.*

When clients call looking for a staff member who is no longer there, it is more difficult to get them back into the salon.

Margo: *Jack, this is Margo from Sensations Salon. I'm calling about your appointment with Thomas next Wednesday. Thomas is leaving to go to another salon, so I would like to reschedule your appointment. We would like to keep your business, Jack, so we are offering your first haircut at half price. John has time for your cut at the same time you were scheduled with Thomas. Would that be all right with you?*

Jack: *Where is Thomas going to be working now?*

Margo: *He is going to be the manager of the hair salon at Madison's Day Spa.*

Jack: *That's the one downtown?*

Margo: *Yes, it is. Do you want the phone number?*

Jack: *Yeah, I do.*

Margo: *It's 555-1111.*

Jack: *Ya know, I think I'll take that appointment with John after all. I really don't want to change unless I have to.*

When clients call looking for a staff member who is no longer there, it is more difficult to get them back into the salon.

Margo: *Good afternoon, Sensations Salon, this is Margo. How can I help you?*

Louise: *I need an appointment next Tuesday, anytime, with Thomas for my color and cut.*

Margo: *Who am I speaking to, please?*

Louise: *This is Louise Pfeiffer.*

Margo: *Oh, hello, Louise. We haven't seen you for a while. Weren't you in Australia for over a month?*

Louise: *Yes, and now I am desperate for color.*

Margo: *Louise, Thomas isn't working here any longer. I can schedule you with Carl, our color technician. You know him, don't you?*

Louise: *Yes, I know Carl. He trained Thomas, didn't he?*

Margo: *You're right, he did. I can schedule you with Carl for your color and Jennifer for your cut. You have been a good customer for a long time and we don't want to lose you. If you schedule today, I can give you half off your haircut. How does that sound?*

Louise: *To be honest, Margo, I would like Thomas to do it for me. Do you know where he is working?*

Margo: *He is at Madison's Day Spa. The phone number is 555-1111.*

Louise: *Thank you, Margo. It is very nice of you to tell me. Oh! What about my color formula? Does he have my formula?*

Margo: *No, he doesn't and I don't believe he is using the same brand of color that we use here.*

Louise: *Do you suppose you could give my color formula to Thomas?*

Margo: *No, I can't do that, but I can give it to you. Hold on while I pull your file.*

(Margo reads the file to Louise.)

Louise: *Thank you so much, Margo. I'm going to miss your salon.*

Margo: *We'll miss you too, Louise. Remember, you're welcome back anytime.*

Traffic Control

The receptionist is generally in charge of all trafficking in the salon. A perusal of the appointment book and a glance at who is seated in the reception area will tell her where to send assistants to help busy stylists. Usually the receptionist has a good idea of what every staff member is doing and to whom at all times.

At Sensations Salon, Jennifer, a stylist, is running thirty minutes behind schedule. Her waiting client is on her lunch break.

Margo: *Mrs. Wright, Jennifer is running behind schedule. I know you are on your lunch break, so if you can't wait for Jennifer, Marc has an opening and could take you right away.*

Mrs. Wright: *I don't know Marc. Is he good?*

Margo: *I'm sure you've seen him many times. Marc's the stylist who works directly behind Jennifer. He is an excellent stylist.*

Mrs. Wright: *I don't know. What other choice do I have?*

Margo: *You could wait till Jennifer gets to you or you could reschedule with her at a later date.*

Mrs. Wright: *Maybe I'll try Marc this time since I'm on my lunch break. Jennifer won't get angry, will she?*

Margo: *No, she is aware that you only have an hour for lunch and it was she who suggested Marc to do your hair. And I know she'll take a second to fill him in on your style.*

(Another client sitting in the reception area suddenly stands and approaches the reception desk.)

Myra: *Did I hear you say that Jennifer is running behind? How long will I have to wait?*

Margo:	Yes, Myra. Jennifer is running a little behind. It will be about thirty minutes before she gets to you. Can I get you some coffee or tea while you are waiting? We just received the new W magazine. Would you like to see it?
Myra:	No, I don't need anything. Do I have time to run to the post office and dry cleaner?
Margo:	That would be a great idea, Myra. Please get back in about twenty minutes and I will have an assistant get you ready for your color.

(Margo immediately gets on the phone to Paul, Jennifer's 1:00 P.M. client.)

Margo:	Hello, Paul. I tried to call you to let you know that Jennifer is running about thirty minutes behind schedule. I hope that isn't going to be too inconvenient for you.
Paul:	Actually, Margo, it is. I have a golf tee time at 2:00 P.M. so a thirty-minute wait won't work.
Margo:	When can we reschedule?

Sometimes a receptionist can take advantage of the time clients must wait for stylists by offering other services, such as a brow arch, a scalp treatment, or a manicure.

Margo:	Good morning, Cynthia. Today you are scheduled to have a facial, right?
Cynthia:	Yes, a facial.
Margo:	Your technician is running a little behind schedule today. How would you like to have a manicure while you're waiting?
Cynthia:	That sounds good. How long will I be here today? I have to pick up my kids at 3:30.
Margo:	No problem, Cynthia. We'll have you finished by three.

Barbara Salomone
Conservatory of Esthetics
Bioelements/Conservatory
of Esthetics
Des Plains, IL

When the stylist or technician is running behind schedule, suggest a complimentary mini-service. One that works well for many salons is a paraffin hand dip. This can satisfy a waiting client for fifteen minutes.

What to Say When Clients Are Late

Mrs. Jones comes rushing into the salon, twenty minutes late. "Oh, Margo," she cries, "my daughter called from Europe just as I was leaving the house. I just had to talk to her. Can I still have my appointment?"

Margo: *Mrs. Jones, let me talk to your stylist to see how we can work this out.* (talks to the stylist and returns to talk to Mrs. Jones) *Twenty minutes is a little too much lost time to go ahead with your appointment. However, Jennifer said she would work you in if you didn't mind waiting in between some other clients. It might take an hour to an hour and a half.*

Mrs. Jones: *Oh, Margo, I can't. I have to get home. My husband is bringing some clients home for dinner.*

Margo: *How about if I check to see if another stylist is available, Mrs. Jones?*

Mrs. Jones: *Could you do that for me?*

The Chronically Late Client

Les Edgerton

Bold Strokes

Ft. Wayne, IN

We have a standard, iron-clad rule. If clients are more than ten minutes late, they have to reschedule and pay in advance for the next visit. We don't tolerate lateness and demand the same respect for time as we give clients.

Every salon has those few clients who are chronically late. You could get to know them and schedule around them. However, as soon as you know you can count on your client being ten minutes late, and you schedule someone else in that slot, your late client will be on time and get upset because another client is in her space. Another option is to confront the client. But be cautious! If you confront a client about his lateness and he mends his ways, be sure you are always on schedule for that client.

Marc's client is twenty minutes late today. The same client has been late for every appointment she has ever had with Marc. Today Marc will confront her about the problem.

Marc: *Connie, your appointment today was at 2:00. It is now 2:20. I have another client due at 2:30 and I can't possibly get your hair done in ten minutes even if I rush through it.*

Wouldn't you rather that I have plenty of time to do your haircut?

Connie: *Yes, I really don't want you to rush my cut. I'm so sorry I'm late. The phone rang just as I was going out the door.*

Marc: *I have to ask you to be on time from now on. If just a few clients are twenty minutes late on a busy day, I can get really far behind schedule, and I hate to run behind.*

Connie: *I'm sorry Marc, I do understand.*

Marc: *Well, all I can do now is work you in between clients. I'll start your cut and then when my next client comes in, I'll stop and take care of her. It will probably be an hour and a half before I have you done.*

Connie: *Oh dear. I'm supposed to meet a friend at three. Is there any other way?*

Marc: *Well, you could have another stylist do your cut today. Or you could reschedule with me for another day. My book is really full right now, so I think you'll have to wait two weeks.*

Connie: *I really don't want anyone but you to cut my hair, Marc. I'll call my friend and tell him I'll be late.*

In another situation, Margo interrupts John, who is drying his client's hair.

Margo: *John, sorry to interrupt you,, but your next client Bob Brown is waiting for you. He would like to know how long you will be.*

John: *Tell him I'll be about fifteen minutes.*

Margo: *OK. But he seems too be a little impatient.*

John: *I've waited for him many times. He can wait for me today.*

(Margo returns to the reception desk and informs Bob that he will have to wait about fifteen minutes for John.)

Bob: *I'm getting more than a little tired of coming in here and waiting. Every time I come in I have to wait at least ten*

Barbara Salomone
Conservatory of Esthetics
Bioelements/Conservatory/
of Esthetics
Des Plains, IL

When the client is too late to do the service at all, reschedule and offer a complimentary makeup touch-up or neck and shoulder massage. Make sure it has been explained to the client that the salon does not want to rush through the service.

Dorothy Floro

Clipps Salon

Pittsburg, PA

For chronically late clients, Dorothy Floro suggests posting a small notice saying, "Please remember that being just ten minutes late inconveniences your stylist and every other client for the rest of the day."

minutes. I make appointments every month, a month in advance, and I always have to wait. I even started coming in late because he was always off schedule. I've had enough. I'll go somewhere else.

Margo: *I understand how you feel. I would feel the same way. We really don't want to lose your business. If I can get someone to cut your hair right now, would you do it?*

Bob: *Depends on who.*

Margo: *Let me look at the book . . . It looks like Diane, the salon manager, has time right now. Diane is an excellent stylist and you could tell her about your problem with John. Would you like to go with Diane?*

Bob: *That would be fine.*

(Later, John approaches Margo and Diane about Bob.)

John: *Explain to me what was going on with Bob. I was only a few minutes late for his appointment, and, besides, he is always late.*

Margo: *He feels that he has been a good client and you have taken advantage of him. He said he has to wait every time he comes in. And he said that he comes in late because he always has to wait anyway, and then you only take about ten minutes to cut his hair.*

Diane: *He was very upset, John. He told me the same thing. In fact, I don't know if he will come back again.*

John: *I have been cutting his hair for at least six years. Maybe I should spend more time with his cut, but, you know, he only has a little bit of hair around the edges now. He always wants it cut exactly the same way. There just isn't that much to do.*

Margo: *Maybe so, John. But he deserves your attention anyway. And I have noticed that you are running behind schedule when Bob comes in. Maybe you could look at the book to see if I should schedule things differently.*

John: *You're right, Margo, I'll call him and apologize.*

Sensations Salon hired an additional receptionist for afternoon and evening duty. Margo is training her. Margo observes as the new receptionist, Beth, answers a call.

Beth: *Good afternoon, Sensations Salon, this is Beth. How can I help you?*

Paul: *I need to make an appointment for a haircut.*

Beth: *With which stylist?*

Paul: *I need it with John for Thursday evening after six.*

Beth: *Sorry, but John doesn't have any openings Thursday night.*

Paul: *Oh, all right. I'll call back another time.*

Beth: *OK. (Beth hangs up the phone.)*

Margo: *Beth, who was that?*

Beth: *It was some man who wanted a haircut with John. But John didn't have time.*

Margo: *You didn't get his name?*

Beth: *No, I didn't.*

Margo: *Next time, get the name first. If they don't offer it, ask them, "Who is calling, please?" Then if you can't get them in when they want, you have to give them options.*

Beth: *Like what?*

Margo: *Like another stylist, another evening, or do they want us to call if there is a cancellation?*

Beth: *That makes sense. I'm sorry. I'll remember next time. There is the phone ringing again. It certainly is busy around here.*

Beth: *Good afternoon, Sensations Salon, this is Beth. How can I help you?*

Lisa: *Hello, Beth. This is Lisa Kent. I need to cancel an appointment I have with John on Thursday.*

Beth: *You mean your cut at 6:15?*

Lisa: *Yes, that's it. Thanks.*

Beth   (hangs up the phone):   *I see now why I need to get clients' names. That man that called earlier could have an appointment with John just when he wanted, if I knew who he was.*

Margo: *Yes, that's right. That kind of thing happens a lot. Remember always to get clients' names. Also, for the client who just canceled, did you suggest that she reschedule right away?*

Beth: *No, I didn't.*

Margo: *If that was Lisa Kent, she always forgets to call and then tries to get in at the last minute. It's important to remind clients to schedule another appointment when they have to cancel. Just say to them, "When would you like to reschedule?" It's as simple as that.*

Beth: *Am I ever going to catch on to this job?*

Margo: *Beth, you have learned much more in these first three days than anyone else I have trained. You are doing a wonderful job.*

Product Returns

Of course, you always handle product returns according to your salon policy. However, to retain clients, it is imperative that the client feels that it is absolutely acceptable to return the product. Even the most loyal client might not come back if she is embarrassed or uncomfortable when returning product. Given the option of losing a good client or losing a few dollars, a salon receptionist sensibly chooses to lose the retail sale.

Mrs. Peters is a long-time client of the salon and uses many of the salon's services. She purchased a brush last time she had her color and cut done. An inappropriate salon dialogue in this situation is as follows:

To retain clients, it is imperative that the client feels that it is absolutely acceptable to return the product.

Margo: *Hello, Mrs. Peters. I don't see you on the appointment schedule. What can I do for you today?*

Mrs. Peters	(hands a package to Margo): *Margo, last week I bought this brush. I really don't like it and I want to return it.*
Margo:	*Oh, I'm so sorry, Mrs. Peters, but used hair brushes aren't returnable.*
Mrs. Peters:	*Well, Monique should have told me that when she sold it to me.*
Margo:	*Yes, she should have told you. However, that doesn't change the salon policy.*
Mrs. Peters:	*But this was a very expensive brush. I don't like the way it feels on my scalp. I really don't want it.*
Margo:	*As I said, Mrs. Peters, we can't take back used hair brushes. I'm sorry.*
Mrs. Peters:	*Well, take it back then without giving me my money back. And cancel my next appointment with Monique.*

A more appropriate salon dialogue would be as follows:

Margo:	*Hello, Mrs. Peters. I don't see you on the appointment schedule. What can I do for you today?*
Mrs. Peters	(hands a package to Margo): *Margo, last week I bought this brush. I really don't like it and I want to return it.*
Margo:	*Oh, Mrs. Peters, we don't usually take returns on hair brushes. Did Monique recommend it for you?*
Mrs. Peters:	*Yes, she did, and she did not say I couldn't return it.*
Margo:	*Mrs. Peters, you are such a good client of our salon, I'm sure we can do something for you. How about if I give you a credit that you can use when you need any hair or skin care products?*
Mrs. Peters:	*That's fine, Margo. Thanks.*

Children in the Salon

Occasionally, clients bring children into the salon. Even if most children in your salon are well-behaved, there are always a few that disrupt stylists and annoy other clients. This can be a sensitive area to confront. Many salons simply do not allow children in the salon unless they are receiving services. However, what about the client whose babysitter cancels at the last minute, so she bundles up her small child and brings her to the salon? After all, she thinks, it's only a half hour or so. If you insist that clients not bring children, you could alienate clients. If you choose to allow children in your salon, it's a good idea to have some distractions on hand to keep children busy until their parents are finished.

If you choose to allow children in your salon, it's a good idea to have some distractions on hand to keep children busy until their parents are finished.

Margo: *Hello, Nora. I see you have your children with you today.*

Nora: *Yes, my sitter canceled at the last minute and I have to get my hair cut before tomorrow. I'm doing a presentation in Seattle Thursday. This could be the biggest sale of my career.*

Margo: *Well congratulations, Nora. John will be with you in just a minute. Did you remember that you are also scheduled for your nails?*

Nora: *Oh no. I forgot. I guess you kids are going to be here longer than I expected.*

Margo: *Let me get them some paper and pencils for drawing.*

Nora: *Thank you, Margo. Now kids, you just stay here in the reception room while I go get my hair and nails done.*

Margo: *Nora, I would prefer that they stay with you. There is a chair near John's station where they can sit. And Nora, please watch them closely. There are all kinds of things in the salon that could harm them. You know, like scissors, razor blades, hot curling irons, things like that.*

Nora: *Oh, OK. Margo. I'll watch them carefully.*

Don't allow the salon receptionist or any staff member to become a babysitter for clients' children. Admittedly, it is impossible for clients to relax when their children need watching. However, it is the client's responsibility to care of her children, not the salon's.

Other people's children can be an irritation to clients, especially if the clients also have young children and have hired a sitter for the day so they can relax at the salon.

Marc: *Hello, Cathy. I see you brought your baby today.*

Cathy: *I didn't want to, but I couldn't find a sitter. She'll be OK. It's her nap time and she'll probably sleep for an hour or so.*

Marc: *Bring her with you. We'll make a space for her by my station.*

(Monique, who works beside Marc, is already cutting her client, Jan.)

Jan: *It is so nice to relax here. I seldom have peace and quiet anymore.*

Monique: *I understand that. With three children, I don't know how you get anything accomplished.*

Marc (brings a freshly shampooed Cathy to his styling chair):
Just put the baby right here in the corner. I think her little carry basket will fit there.

Cathy: *Perfect. I'm glad she is sleeping so soundly.*

Marc: *So am I.*

(At the other side of the salon, John turns on his blow dryer, which immediately wakens Cathy's baby. The baby begins to cry.)

Cathy: *Don't worry about it, Marc. She will cry herself back to sleep in a minute or two.*

Jan: *Oh no. I can't stand to hear that baby cry. I came here to relax. Can't you do something, Monique?*

Monique: *I don't know what to do. Wait a minute and see if she stops crying.*

Jan: *Monique, I know that cry. She isn't going to stop anytime soon.*

(Monique uses strong body language to tell Marc: "Please do something.")

Dwight Miller

Anasazi Exclusive Products

Dubuque, IA

To retain clients, be sure you get them thinking about what's going to happen next time. Plan small changes in the haircut or perm so the client will have something to look forward to. Also, teach clients a little at a time. I've learned that about teaching scalp massage. If you teach them too many manipulations to do, they do nothing. If you give them another step every time they come to your salon, they will learn and follow through better.

Marc:	*Cathy, I think your baby is disturbing other clients. Can you quiet her?*
Cathy	(picks up her baby): *I'll try. Maybe I should walk around with her and try to get her back to sleep.*
Marc:	*OK, but I have another client in half an hour. Your hair is partially cut, so I'll have to finish it.*
Cathy:	*I'll be just a minute.*
Monique:	*Marc, crying babies really upset everyone. Can you have her go someplace else?*
Marc:	*Like where? I don't like crying babies either, you know.*
Monique:	*She is crying even louder now, Marc. Send her home!*
Marc:	*Cathy, why don't you take your baby home? You can come back later, maybe when your husband can watch her. That way you can relax and be sure to get a good haircut. With the baby crying, I can't concentrate anyway.*
Cathy:	*Marc, I can't go home with half a haircut!*
Marc:	*You can come back today. I'll even stay late tonight to get you finished.*
Cathy:	*I guess I don't have a choice, do I?*

(Cathy bundles up her crying baby and leaves the salon.)

Jan:	*Thank you, Monique. I really wish you had a specific policy about bringing children here. If you hadn't done something about her, I was going to look for another hairdresser.*
Monique:	*Well, in that case, Jan, I'm glad Marc handled it the way he did.*

Checking Out

The script for clients leaving the salon is as important as the dialogue when they enter the salon. To move clients through the checkout procedure with a minimum of fuss and confusion, create step-by-step procedures for client checkout.

Sensations Salon has a specific client checkout procedure:

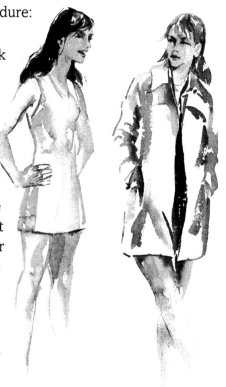

- The attending staff member walks to the reception desk with the client.
- The staff member gives the completed client file to the receptionist.
- The staff member locates the recommended retail products for the client.
- The staff member says, "Thank you (client's name), I look forward to seeing you next time. Margo will take care of you at the desk and get your next appointment scheduled. Good-bye." The stylist gives the client over to the receptionist, saying, "(Client's name) will need an appointment for (recommended services) in _____ weeks."
- The receptionist schedules future appointments, mentions the current salon promotions, and then takes money for the service and retail.

Scheduling Ahead

When the client is at the desk ready to check out, the first step in the exiting procedure is to schedule the client's next appointment.

Karen is at the reception desk waiting to pay for her services.

Margo: *Hello, Karen. Your new cut looks great. You're wearing it longer now, aren't you?*

Karen: *Thanks, Margo. I like it, too.*

Margo: *Will you need your next color and cut in five weeks or six?*

Karen: *Probably six now that it's a little longer.*

Margo: *Is six weeks from now at the same time convenient with you?*

Karen: *That should be. Let me look at a calendar. No, that isn't good. I'll be on vacation then. How about a week earlier?*

Margo: *OK. Same time?*

Karen: *Yes, 5:30 is good.*

Margo: *Your appointment is at 5:30 on Wednesday, June 22nd, for a color, cut, and style. Should I use the same phone number to confirm?*

Karen: *Yes, that's my home phone. Just leave a message on my recorder.*

When the Client Doesn't Schedule

Some clients find it difficult to schedule their appointments more than a week or two ahead. If you are a stylist who is booked solid six weeks in advance, you don't have to be concerned with clients who don't schedule ahead. However, stylists who are developing a client base should do all they can to get their clients back into the salon on schedule. Some suggestions are as follows:

Send reminder cards to clients ten days or two weeks before they are due for a service.

Offer to call clients to remind them to schedule.

Suggest that clients make a note on their calendar to call for an appointment on a certain date.

Remind clients that it is better to schedule in advance, especially when they have a pressured lifestyle and might find it difficult to get an appointment when it's convenient for them.

Purchasing Products

If the attending salon professional fails to get clients' retail products for them, the receptionist should be sure to check clients' files or the computer files to see what products they have purchased in the past. Asking "Do you need any shampoo?" requires a closed yes or no answer. A better approach would be, "Which products did your stylist (or technician) recommend for you?" or

"How do you like the Therma Shampoo you have been using? You are probably almost finished with that 8-ounce bottle you purchased last time. Would you like to buy a larger one this time?"

This is also an ideal time to inform clients about special offers in retail. Look for product specials that will fit your clients' hair and lifestyle. For example, "We have a special right now on leave-in conditioner with sunscreen. If you buy a 32-ounce bottle, you get a 4-ounce travel size for free. It's just the right size to take to the beach. It's just as important to protect your hair from the sun as it is to protect your skin." A male client who gets a very short haircut every three weeks would not be as interested in this special offer as a female client with long, highlighted hair.

Margo: *You are probably running out of your Thermprotection Shampoo. Would you like to buy the larger size this time? It's more economical, and you won't run out so soon. Besides, we're having a special on it right now. If you buy a 32-ounce shampoo, you can get an 8-ounce styling lotion for half price.*

Karen: *You're right, I am running out of shampoo, and that sounds like a good deal. I also need some hairspray. I haven't used your hairspray before. Which one do you recommend?*

Margo: *We have three types: working spray that is very light, a medium hold, and a firm hold.*

Karen: *I'll take the light hold.*

Margo: *Is there anything else I can get for you, Karen?*

Karen: *I think that's it.*

Inform clients about special offers in retail. Look for product specials that will fit your clients' hair and lifestyle.

Collecting the Payment

Ask clients about their method of payment. For example, "Will that be cash, check, or charge?" To avoid making mistakes when giving change to clients, be sure to count it out for them. When you offer clients a receipt, also give them any written material, such as salon newsletters, special offers they might be able to use, as well as the written salon guarantee.

The Guarantee

Before you end the exiting dialogue—perhaps while you are bagging up the products—remind clients of your guarantee.

Margo: *Remember, Karen, that all our services are guaranteed. If you are unhappy about anything we did, please call us right away. There is a copy of our guarantee in the salon brochure that I put in your bag.*

Thank You

The final step in the exiting procedure is to thank clients for their business.

Margo: *Thank you, Karen. We appreciate your business. See you next month.*

Karen: *Bye, Margo.*

Chapter Summary

1. Society has become so used to customization we must also customize the way we schedule appointments. All of our clients are different, with various demands for several types of perming services and a multitude of coloring services.

2. To complicate scheduling procedures for a receptionist, salon personnel work at different rates. Inexperienced personnel usually require additional time for services, while accomplished personnel all work at different speeds.

3. The receptionist is generally in charge of all trafficking in the salon. A glance at the appointment book and another at who is seated in the reception area will tell her where to send assistants to help busy stylists.

4. Every salon has clients who are chronically late. You could get to know them and schedule around them; however, the best solution is to deal with them in a straightforward fashion.

5. Handle product returns according to your salon policy. To retain clients, it is imperative that the client feels that it is absolutely acceptable to return the product. Even the most loyal client might not come back if she is embarrassed or uncomfortable when returning product.

6. Occasionally, clients bring children into the salon. Even if most children in your salon are well-behaved, there are always a few that disrupt stylists and annoy other clients. This can be a sensitive issue to confront, but it is crucial when considering the clients who are discomforted by unruly children.

7. The script for clients leaving the salon is as important as the dialogue when they enter the salon. To move clients through the checkout procedure with a minimum of fuss and confusion, create step-by-step procedures for client checkout.

Chapter

8

The Prospective Client

For the most part, the phone is your first contact with a prospective client. Those first few seconds on the phone create a first impression based on which the prospect will decide whether or not you were friendly, helpful, courteous, or efficient and will make a host of other judgments simply by the way you speak. After the initial greeting, you must find out if the person on the other end of the line is a new prospect or an established client. Callers give us many clues to tell us that they are new customers, but if there is any doubt, simply ask ("Have you been to our salon before?" or "Are you new to our salon?"). A prospective client must be handled differently and asked different questions than a regular salon client.

Janet: *Good morning. Sensations Salon. This is Janet. How can I help you?*

Prospect: *Yes, Janet. I would like to have a haircut appointment with Jackie.*

Janet: *OK. May I have your name, please?*

Prospect: *Yes, this is Bob Cromroy.*

Janet: *Bob. We don't have a Jackie here. Is it possible you meant Jennifer?*

Bob: *Could be. I want whoever cuts Jim Harden's hair.*

When Bob didn't have the correct name of a stylist, Janet realized right away that Bob was either a new prospect or hadn't been to the salon often. Janet also knew that she needed to have the customer's name before making an issue out of remembering a stylist's name. Janet built rapport with Bob by using his name.

Janet: *Bob, hold on for just a minute while I look up Jim Harden's file. . . . That's Jennifer. She has an opening tomorrow at 1 P.M. Is that convenient for you?*

Bob: *It sure is. I'll be on my lunch hour, though. Does she usually run on schedule?*

Janet: *Tomorrow's schedule looks fairly easy. I don't think she'll be running behind. However, if something does make her run behind schedule, I'll call you right away. Is there a phone number where I can reach you?*

Just a few sentences can give the prospect clues about the professionalism of a salon. Bob is impressed that Janet will take time to be sure he is scheduling with the right stylist and that she will call him if his stylist is running behind.

Bob: *My work number is 555-1234. If I'm out of the office, leave a message on my voice mail. I check it regularly.*

Janet: *Thank you, Bob. Do you know where we are located?*

Bob: *As a matter of fact, I do. Jim told me how to get there.*

Janet: *Great. I'll see you tomorrow at 1 P.M. for your haircut with Jennifer. Thank you, Bob. Good-bye.*

Be sure to ask if the new prospect knows your salon location. A new prospect arriving at your salon frustrated and anxious is no way to start a relationship, and there are few things more frustrating than being late for an appointment because you can't find the location of the salon.

There are three ways that new prospects hear about your salon:

1. They were referred by another client.
2. They were attracted by your advertising.
3. They were referred by a manufacturer of a product you use.

Client Referrals

When a client refers someone to your salon, chances are the prospective customer wants to use the same stylist as his or her friend. The prospect already has a preconceived good image of your salon created by the referring friend. Scheduling should be easy because the prospect already knows which stylist he or she wants The only thing left to do in scheduling is to find out the desired service and service time.

Advertising Referrals

When prospective clients appear at your door because they were attracted by your advertising, they don't have a stylist in mind. Their concept of your salon is the image created by your advertising. In this case, ideally the receptionist should question prospective clients to fit them with the best possible stylist for their hair and personality type.

Margo: *Since you aren't familiar with our salon, I would like to ask you a few questions so we can get you with the stylist who would work best with you. Do you wear your hair longer than chin length?*

Sally: *Yes. It's almost to my shoulder, but I want a good deal of it cut off.*

Margo: *OK. Do you like a more trendy look or do you prefer conservative styles, Sally?*

Sally: *Actually, I think you could describe it as casual. I don't like to fuss with it. I need a simple style that takes a minimum of work. I just don't have extra time in the mornings.*

Les Edgerton

Bold Strokes

Fort Wayne, IN

We ask clients to send us their best friend. We're all booked solid for six to eight weeks. I've worked all over the country, in all kinds of situations, and have always been booked like that.

Margo: What kind of work do you do, Sally?

Sally: Oh, I'm in sales for a medical supply company. Could I have an appointment Thursday evening? I'm gong out of town Friday.

Margo: I think you would like John to style your hair. He has an opening at 7:15 Thursday. How does that sound?

Sally: That would be just fine.

Margo: Sally, since this is your first time in our salon, would you please come in ten minutes early to fill out our new client questionnaire?

Sally: Sure, I'll be there.

Margo: Now all I need is your phone number.

Manufacturer Referrals

In recent years, manufacturers have discovered the benefits of a referral service, in which they direct consumer calls to salons nearest the caller. With the growing popularity of infomercials, many consumers calling to order professional products are directed to professional salons that carry the manufacturer's products.

When you get a manufacturer's referral, you know the prospect already uses professional products and probably is conscientious about hair and skin care. An alert receptionist can qualify the caller to find a good stylist match when the client doesn't know which stylist he or she wants.

Acknowledge clients as soon as they enter your reception area. If you wait longer than ten seconds, clients begin to feel uncomfortable. Acknowledging simply means letting customers know that you are aware of their presence. If the reception desk is busy with phone calls and clients, the acknowledgment can be in the form of a simple nod of the head or wave of the hand.

If you are the first person to greet customers, call them by name and confirm their service, appointment time, and stylist.

It's a busy day at Sensations Salon. Margo, the receptionist, is on the phone scheduling an appointment. Another line rings and a customer walks in the door. Margo makes eye contact with the entering client and waves hello. When the call is finished, she addresses the customer.

Margo: *Hi, can I help you?*

Betsy: *Yes. I have an appointment with Marc.*

Margo: *You must be Betsy Tipps. This is your first time here, isn't it?*

Betsy: *Yes, it is.*

Margo: *Welcome to our salon, Betsy. Your appointment is for a perm and cut at eleven. I'm glad you came a little early. We have a questionnaire to fill out before Marc sees you.*

Betsy: *My appointment is at 10:45, and I didn't necessarily want a perm today. When I called I said that I wanted to talk to someone about the possibility of a perm. My hair is color-treated and I don't know if I should perm it.*

Margo: *Oh. I guess we made a mistake. I'll correct it on Marc's schedule. Please complete this questionnaire and Marc will be ready for your consultation in just a few minutes. Can I get you some coffee, tea, or water, Betsy?*

Betsy: *Water would be great, thanks.*

Margo: *If you would like to look at style books, just get some from the magazine rack to the left of the reception chairs. If you want a magazine, those are in the rack on the other side.*

Acknowledge clients as soon as they enter your reception area.

Betsy: *Thanks, maybe looking at some pictures would help me decide what I want to do with my hair.*

(Betsy finishes the questionnaire and returns it to Margo.)

Margo: *Thank you, Betsy. Here is our salon brochure and price list. It has a list of all our services as well as a description of our spa packages.*

Betsy: *I didn't realize you did so many different things. I'll have to show this to my husband.*

Client Orientation

Touring the Salon

The more comfortable prospective clients are with their surroundings, the more likely that they will return. Taking them on a tour of your salon will orient them quickly as well as educate them about your services.

Robert: *Hello, Betsy. I'm Robert. It will be about five more minutes until Marc is ready for you. While you are waiting, I'll show you around the salon. Come with me and I'll show you the spa area first.*

Betsy: *Great. I'd love to see it.*

Robert: *First we'll go upstairs, where we have body massage and treatments. Have you ever had a body polish?*

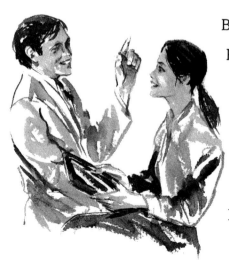

Betsy: *I've had a massage. Is it similar?*

Robert: *No. A polish is a treatment where your entire body is rubbed first with oil and then with an herb that exfoliates your skin. After that, a cream is applied that dissolves the herb. Your skin feels like baby skin afterward.*

Betsy: *Wow. I could really use that in the winter when my skin is dry all over.*

Robert: *Yes, and it's also great before applying any self-tanner, which we also offer as a service. You see, when your skin is exfoliated, your tan looks better.*

Betsy: *Now that you say that, I remember reading about it in a magazine.*

Robert: *This is our body treatment room, and the room next door is pedicure and reflexology. The room is in use now, so maybe I can show it to you later.*

Betsy: *Reflexology fascinates me. I have a friend who has it done regularly, and she swears by it.*

Robert: *Our reflexologist is busy most of the time. I think she is probably the best in this area. Let's go downstairs now and I'll show you our perm and color area.*

(When the tour is over, Betsy feels very comfortable with the salon. She now has seen all the service areas, met some of the staff, and knows where to get coffee or tea if she wants it.)

Robert: *I think Marc is ready for you now. Come with me and I'll take you to his styling chair.*

Taking clients on a tour of the salon will orient them quickly as well as educate them about the services.

Meeting the Stylist or Technician

Often you have just thirty minutes to build enough rapport with prospective clients to make them want to return a second time. The best way to jump start that rapport is to greet prospective clients with a warm smile, a firm handshake, and good eye contact.

A good rapport-building greeting would be, "Good morning, Jackie. I'm John, your stylist," (handshake, eye contact, and smile). "May I get you coffee or tea before we get started?"

Prospective clients are looking for a new stylist and a new salon. Some of the qualities they look for in a stylist are competence, integrity, and reliability. The more you express these qualities, the more likely they will become clients of your salon.

Even on days when you have been working nonstop for hours and you are running behind schedule, it is important to take a few seconds to center yourself before approaching a new client. Prepare yourself to show all your best qualities in your voice and body language.

Today, Jennifer is anything but centered as she approaches her new client.

(Margo pages Jennifer for the third time.)

Margo: *Jennifer, your next client is here.*

Jennifer (appears at the reception desk): *Oh, hi there. Would you please have a seat in my styling chair? Uh . . . it's the third from the left. I'll be right back. Gotta take a potty break.*

(Jennifer's new customer wanders around the salon looking for something that might be Jennifer's chair. She finally chooses an empty chair and sits down.)

Jennifer: *Oh no! Not that chair—this one over here.* (Jennifer waves to her client to come to the other end of the salon.)

Jennifer: *Here it is. Just have a seat. What can I do for you? What was your name again?*

Karen: *My name is Karen. Are you Jennifer?*

Jennifer: *Yeah, I'm Jennifer. How do you want your hair cut?*

Karen: *I'm not sure. Do you have any ideas?*

Jennifer: *Well, I only have half an hour. Why don't you get it the same this time and we'll change it next time? You could come in a few minutes earlier and look at style books. How does that sound?*

Karen: *OK. I guess I could do that.*

Is it surprising that Karen never rebooked with Jennifer?

Quality, Service, and Expertise

To draw a constant stream of new clients into your salon, you must have an excellent salon image and offer great value to your clients. Value is the balance of quality, expertise, and service as weighed against the cost in dollars. Your body language enhances value—the way you handle products—whereas your words and actions demonstrate your expertise.

To demonstrate your expertise through your words, be a problem solver for the client. For example, "You say that your hair is always flat. Did you know that if there is just a slight bit of layering your hair wouldn't be quite so heavy and, additionally, we have a shampoo that will remove all the debris from your hair that could be weighing it down? Let me show you."

You can't be a problem solver unless you know the features and benefits of your services and products or if you don't have the technical knowledge to understand what the hair needs.

Prospective Client Fears

Most prospective clients are in your chair because they were recommended by a friend. However, just because you please their friend doesn't mean you will satisfy them. Most prospective clients are apprehensive. Often all they can think about is the worst experience they ever had at a salon and wonder if this one will be he same. Circling in their minds are thoughts such as the following:

Perhaps the hairstylist will cut my hair too short.

The nail technician could burn my nails with the drill during sculptured nail fill.

The pedicurist might not use sanitary instruments and I could get an infection.

What if the color technician turns my hair green or brassy?

What if I'm allergic to the skin treatment and I turn red or break out in a rash?

Most prospective clients are apprehensive. Often all they can think about is the worst experience they ever had at a salon.

It's important to identify prospective clients' fears and dispel them.

Marc: *Betsy, Margo said you wanted to talk to me about getting a perm. Is that right?*

Betsy: *Yes. I would love to have more body in my hair, but I'm afraid my hair will be damaged if I perm it.*

Marc: *How long has it been since you had a perm?*

Betsy: *It's been about fifteen years. I think I was a teenager when I had my last perm.*

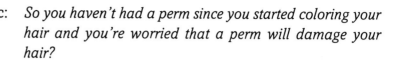

Marc: *So you haven't had a perm since you started coloring your hair and you're worried that a perm will damage your hair?*

Betsy: *Right. I like my hair to be soft and natural looking. I've seen a lot of people with fried perms, and I couldn't tolerate my hair looking like that. But I really would like to have some movement in my hair. It just hangs there, and even if I curl it the curl only lasts for an hour. What should I do?*

Marc: *Your hair has great texture, and I love your auburn color. Anytime you put chemical on your hair, you get a certain amount of damage; however, you have very strong hair that will perm wonderfully. There won't be any noticeable damage if you get your hair permed. You will have just great body and fullness.*

Betsy: *You promise?*

Marc: *I guarantee it.*

Betsy: *OK, let's do it.*

Client Retention

We could call the prospective customer a new client except that people do not become clients until they come back at least five times. It takes that long for people to accept you as their hairdresser. If you check your client retention rates, you might find that 70% of prospective customers never make it to the fifth visit. Typically what happens is that on the first visit the stylist or technician is very attentive to the client. The stylist takes time to consult with the client, listens to her needs, and makes sure that she is comfortable.

John: *Hello, Susan. My name is John and I am going to be your stylist today. Before we get started, I'd like to take you around the salon to show you where everything is located.*

Then I would like to take a few minutes to talk with you about your hair before it is shampooed.

(After the salon tour, John takes Susan to his styling chair.)

John: *Would you like some coffee, tea, or water before we get started?*

Susan: *I'd really like some coffee. Do you have decaf?*

John: *Yes, we do, Susan. How do you take it?*

(John brings coffee to Susan and proceeds to do a thorough consultation. Afterward, he cuts and styles her hair.)

John (holds the hand mirror for Susan to see her hair): *Let me show you your style from all sides and I'll recap what has been done. First I used our clarifying shampoo to remove all the residue that weighs down your hair. Then I used a very light surface-active rinse. Your hair is healthy, so you can stop using those heavy conditioners you have at home. You need just a very light leave-in spray condition. Next I used about five pumps of spray glaze* (hands her the bottle) *to give your hair body, and I finished your hair with our finishing spray* (hands her the bottle). *To get this fullness on top, use your brush to lift at the scalp area, just like I showed you. Does all that make sense, or should I review it again?*

Susan: *No, I think I have it, John. You did a great job. I love it!*

If you check your client retention rates, you might find that 70% of prospective customers never make it to the fifth visit.

On the second visit, John also does a great job of making Susan happy. However, when Susan returns for the third visit, John is running behind schedule and Susan has to wait twenty-five minutes. She hasn't had to wait before, so this time waiting is acceptable. When John finally gets to Susan, he takes her straight to the shampoo bowl without even looking at her asking her how her haircut was working out. Again Susan excuses John because she sees that he has a very busy day. However, the following day Susan realizes that this haircut is a little too short on top. Susan makes a mental note to tell John about it next time she gets a haircut.

On her fourth visit, Susan again must wait; however, this time it's only about fifteen minutes. When John takes Susan to the shampoo area, she stops him. "I need to show you something about this haircut before you shampoo me. I'd like to have it cut the way you did it the first time."

"Oh, OK," he says in an irritated voice. "Can you wait a minute while I check on a color I have processing? I'll just be a second. Go sit in my styling chair until I get back."

During Susan's consultation and service time, John leaves her three times to check his color client. Every time he comes back, Susan wonders if he knows where he left off in her haircut. She becomes even more agitated when he parts her hair on the wrong side. This time when Susan leaves the salon, she doesn't schedule her next cut. "I'll call," she says.

Often salon personnel begin to take the client for granted after the second visit or, even worse, not remember the client at all. Either way, there is a good chance of losing the client. Often by the fourth visit (if the prospect makes it to the fourth visit), the stylist will not put as much effort into the service as on the first or second visit. If during the first and second visit you treat the prospect like a queen, on the third you treat her like a special person, and on the fourth you barely talk to her but you just do the same haircut as the previous three times and you don't remember her kids' names or where she has relocated from, you are in danger of losing the client.

Often salon personnel begin to take the client for granted after the second visit or, even worse, not remember the client at all.

Ideally, you should use the same procedure every time you see a client. Always treat clients as courteously as the first time, and you will retain them. In addition, the following tips will help you retain clients:

1. Always apologize for making a client wait, even if it is only five minutes. Just a simple "I hope you haven't been waiting long" tells clients that you value their time.

2. Always reconfirm the desired style. Whether it is a new customer or a client who has been around for years, it is extremely important to be sure of the style you are cutting. For example, Monique has already started cutting Sandy's hair when Sandy says, "Monique, you do remember that I wanted to grow out the back of my hair, don't you?"

Monique: *Oh dear, I'm so sorry, Sandy. I forgot. I cut the back off like you used to wear it. I don't know what I was thinking.*

Sandy: *Monique, I have been growing that for three months. How could you forget?*

3. Make a plan for the future. It is important to have a plan for prospective clients through at least five visits to create incentives for the prospect to come back.

John: *I really like this cut on you, Peggy. What would make it better is to grow out this fringe area and crown a little. We can gradually work at it during the next couple of haircuts until it's grown out. Next time, though, it will be time to highlight your hair. A little more highlighting around your eyes would really make your eyes stand out. You should schedule that before you leave today. You could wait until your next cut, or you can get it done within the next few weeks if you want.*

4. Always follow up with new prospects.

John   (on the phone a week later):   *Hello, Peggy. This is John at Sensations Salon. How is your new cut working for you?*

Peggy: *It's great, John. And I can't wait to get my highlighting. I have an appointment for next week.*

John: *Wonderful, I'll see you next week then.*

Follow-Up Calls

To strengthen your relationship and tell your prospective clients that you really care, call them a few days after their service to find out how the style is working and get feedback on their salon visit.

You can also head off any problems by letting clients know it's all right to complain.

Carolyn   (on the phone):   *Hello, this is Carolyn from Sensations Salon. May I speak to Ruth Wagner please?*

Ruth: *Hello, Carolyn, this is Ruth.*

Carolyn: *Hi, Ruth. I'm calling to find out how you are doing with your new set of nails. I know this is the first time you have worn sculptured nails and I want to be sure that you are getting along with them.*

Ruth: *I'm glad you called. I love my nails, but I am having a very difficult time with them. They seem to always be in the way.*

Carolyn: *There is a transition period to go through. After all, this is the first time in your life you've had nails.*

Ruth: *It's more than that. I think you were right about the length. I should have listened to you and had them done shorter.*

Carolyn: *Come into the salon and I'll reshape them for you. I have time late this afternoon.*

Ruth: *I can file them myself, can't I?*

Carolyn: *Yes, you could; however, I would prefer that you come to the salon for that until you are more comfortable with your nails. Additionally, there's a certain way to reshape them so that they look natural, and you do want them to look natural, don't you?*

Ruth: *Yes, you're right, Carolyn. You say you have time this afternoon?*

Check-up calls (or follow-up calls) are a value-added service that can significantly increase your return rate on prospective clients. They are an important method of staying in touch with prospects and a gentle reminder that you are truly a salon professional, concerned about your clients.

Carl, the color technician, is calling Thea, a first-time client who transferred in from another state. Carl had to match the color she has worn for several years. Although Thea brought a formula from her previous hairdresser, it was in a different color brand than Carl used, so he had to reformulate.

Carl: *Hello, Thea. This is Carl from Sensations Salon. How are you today?*

Thea: *Hi there, Carl. I'm fine. What can I do for you?*

Carl: *I'm calling to find out how you like your haircolor.*

Thea: *Oh, you're the stylist who colored my hair! For a minute there I didn't connect who you were.*

Carl: *Yes, I should have explained who I am. After all, you were only in our salon one time. How do you like your color?*

Thea: *Basically the color is fine.*

Carl: *I get the feeling that it could have been better.*

Thea: *Well, yes. I think it used to have more highlights in it.*

Carl: *Do you mean it had lighter strands?*

Thea: *Yes, that's it. And it had many different colors in it. The color you did is kind of flat looking.*

Carl: *When are you available to come in so I can adjust it for you?*

Thea: *Don't worry about it, Carl. I'm too busy to get back in there. The color is fine the way it is. I'm sure that next time you can adjust it.*

Carl: *OK, Thea, I'll make a note on your file to adjust your color next time. I'll see you then in, what, about four weeks?*

Thea: *That's right, I get my color every five weeks.*

Carl: *I can schedule that for you right now, if you like.*

Thea: *Sure, let's do that.*

Prospects become clients when rapport is established as a foundation to a good relationship, when clients are comfortable in your salon, and when they have returned at least five times. Try to relate to your prospects' feelings by remembering how uncomfortable you are when you are in an unfamiliar place. When prospects leave your salon feeling like they are the most important customer you have had all day, they will return, even if the service they received was not exactly what they had in mind.

Chapter Summary

1. The salon phone is your first contact with a prospective client. Those first few seconds on the phone create a first impression based on which the prospect will decide whether or not you were friendly, helpful, courteous, or efficient and will make a host of other judgments simply by the way you speak.

2. There are three ways that new prospects hear about your salon: They were referred by another client; they were attracted by your advertising; or they were referred by a manufacturer of a product you use.

3. Acknowledging clients means letting them know that you are aware of their presence. If the reception desk is busy with phone calls and clients, the acknowledgment can be in the form of a simple nod of the head or wave of the hand.

4. The more comfortable prospective clients are with their surroundings, the more likely that they will return. Taking them on a tour of your salon will orient them quickly as well as educate them about your services.

5. Usually you have only thirty minutes to build enough rapport with prospective clients to make them want to return a second time. The best way to jump start that rapport is to greet prospective clients with a warm smile, a firm handshake, and good eye contact.

6. Most prospective clients are apprehensive and worry that this could be the worst experience they ever had at a salon. Make prospects feel more secure by identifying their fears and dispelling them.

7. To draw a constant stream of new clients into your salon, you must have an excellent salon image and offer great value to your clients. Value is the balance of quality, expertise, and service as weighed against the cost in dollars.

8. We could call the prospective customer a new client except that people do not become clients until they come back at least five times. It takes that long for people to accept you as their hairdresser.

9. You should use the same procedure every time you see a client. Always treat clients as courteously as the first time and you will retain them.

10. To strengthen your relationship and tell your prospective clients that you really care, call them a few days after their service to find out how the style is working and get feedback on their salon visit.

Chapter 9

Consultations

Janet   (approaches her next client from the reception area): *Maxine. Hi there. My name is Janet. I'm going to be in charge of your services today. Come with me to my styling chair and we'll talk for a few minutes.*

Maxine: *I thought Carl was going to color my hair.*

Janet: *Yes, he is, and we'll get him in just a minute. I'm going to style your hair afterward, so before your hair is wet, I want to see how you wear it.*

Maxine: *That's a great idea. I can't tell you how many times I have been rushed through a salon. I've been shampooed before anybody even saw what I looked like and then I have to try to explain my hair to them. This is much better. See how the front of my hair goes? I like it just like that.*

Janet: *OK, Maxine, I think I have it. You like the sides going toward your face, right?*

Maxine: *Yes, I do, and I like the back smooth and neat.*

Edie Noppenberger

Edies's Style Center

Clearwater, FL

Because every client's hair is different, the first critical step in perming is the client consultation. It's impossible to get creative results by using the same perm on every client. You need to determine the hair's porosity, density, elasticity, and texture, since each of these characteristics will affect the way the hair and the chemicals interact during the perm service.

Janet: *Sides, top, back, I got it. Now, your hair looks a little dry. Could I do treatment on it today after your color?*

Maxine: *Conditioners always make my hair limp. I'd rather have dry hair than limp hair.*

Janet: *What if I could give you shiny, healthy hair that is full of body?*

Maxine: *That would be wonderful, but I don't believe it.*

Janet: *Maxine, I have a treatment that is really going to surprise you. I guarantee it.*

Maxine: *By that do you mean that if I don't like it, I don't have to pay for it?*

Janet: *That's right, Maxine.*

Maxine: *All right, you can give me a treatment. Does that happen before or after color?*

Janet: *We could do it either way, but I prefer after. Right now, I want to have you change into a gown for your color. Come with me and I'll show you our changing room.*

Consulting is the process of discovery in which the stylist observes, studies, and detects what the client needs. Its purpose is also to reveal problems that clients might not be aware of, such as hair breakage, product buildup, dry, frizzy hair, or mismatched color.

Using a client questionnaire will enhance consultations. It saves stylists and technicians time, answers many pertinent questions, and gives the stylist openings for additional questions that could improve the overall results of the client's service.

Preshampoo Consultation

Because clients are more comfortable talking to stylists when their hair is dry, establishing rapport with clients is easier when you offer a preshampoo consultation. At the same time, notice the client's body shape, mode of dress, and the way the client has combed her hair.

Monique: *Hello, Joan. I am Monique and I'm going to cut your hair today. I want to take a quick look before Robert shampoos you. Did you have something specific in mind for your cut?*

(Monique examines Joan's current style and then brushes her hair to feel for texture, pliability, and thickness.)

Joan: *Not really. I just want to do something that will give my hair more body.*

Monique: *Were you thinking about going shorter?*

Joan: *I don't know. What did you have in mind?*

Monique: *There are several options. How about if you get shampooed and then we'll discuss all the different cuts we can do on you?*

Joan: *Great.*

Monique: *This is Robert. He will take you to the shampoo area.*

The Shampoo Consultation

A shampoo is an enjoyable, relaxing experience for most people. On the other hand, for people who are ultrasensitive to heat and cold or have tender scalps, the shampoo can be stressful. During a quick consultation with clients, you can find out if they like a firm or gentle massage, warm or cool water, and one or two shampoos and whether or not they have sensitive scalps.

Monique's client has been escorted to the shampoo area.

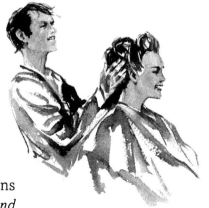

Robert: *Joan, before I shampoo you, I'm going to brush your hair and scalp. Do you like to have it brushed vigorously or more gently?*

Joan: *Oh, please brush it gently. I have a sensitive scalp.*

Robert: *Do you also like your shampoo massage to be gentle?*

Joan: *Well, you could be more firm with the shampoo. I don't like my hair pulled, but I do like to have my head rubbed.*

Robert: *OK, gentle brushing and firm shampoo.* (Robert begins brushing Joan's hair.) *Your hair is color treated and a little on the fine side. Does it go flat soon after it's styled?*

Joan: *Yes, it does. I really envy people who have body in their hair. Mine just hangs all the time, no matter how I get it cut. Oh, that reminds me. Don't use any conditioner, it just makes it worse.*

Robert: *I understand what you mean about your hair going limp. We have many clients with that same problem. I have a shampoo that will build strength in your hair. It's called Wheat Strengthening Shampoo. The treatment that goes with it is especially designed for fine hair. It has no oils in it that can weigh hair down.*

Joan: *Please go ahead and use the shampoo but not the conditioner.*

Robert: *It isn't a conditioner, Joan. I was talking about a treatment for fine hair that is left in. It builds body like you have never seen. Monique will tell you about it when she cuts your hair. For now you'll get a firm shampoo with no conditioner, right?*

Joan: *Right.*

Robert: *Lean back now into the shampoo bowl. Are you comfortable?*

Joan: *Yes, that feels good.*

Robert: *Just another question or two and I'll let you relax. Do you like one or two shampoos and warm or cool water?*

Joan: *Warm water and just one shampoo, please.*

(Robert shampoos Joan and escorts her to Monique's styling chair.)

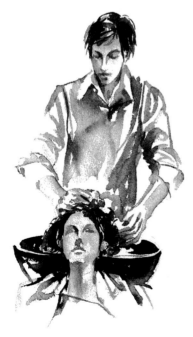

Monique: *Hello, Joan. I see Robert shampooed you. Doesn't he do a wonderful shampoo?*

Joan: *Yes, it was just great. He has a nice touch.*

Be sure clients are comfortable during consultations. It can be difficult for them to stay in good humor if their backs are wet or water is dripping down their faces. Offer them coffee, tea, or other refreshments available at your salon. Review and discuss clients' comments on the questionnaire.

Monique removes the tangles from Joan's hair and begins to analyze Joan's hair and features. Using the client information form that Joan completed when she was in the reception area, Monique proceeds to consult with her new client. Monique comments on some of Joan's responses.

Question: *How did you learn of us?*

Monique: *I see you are a friend of Helen Watts. She is truly a lovely lady, isn't she? I must thank her for recommending you to me. I'm thrilled that so many people use our referral program here. Did you know that if you send three of your friends to me I will send you a gift certificate for a free haircut?*

Clients should be made comfortable during consultations. It can be difficult for them if their backs are wet or water's dripping down their face.

Joan: *What a great idea. Does Helen get a free haircut now?*

Monique: *I don't know. I'll have to pull her file to find out. Before you leave today I will give you some referral cards so you can get a free haircut, too.*

Joan: *Sounds good to me.*

Question: *How often have you visited a salon in the past?*

Monique: *You get your hair cut about once a month? I guess that means you like to keep it about the same length all the time.*

Joan: *It's not that my hair gets too long, it just seems to get out of control so easily.*

Question: *Have you ever had a permanent wave? Within the past year?*

Often a client thinks that if she got a perm a year ago it is gone from her hair. If her hair is more than six inches long, the

New Client Information Form

Today's Date _____

Name _____

Address _____

City_____

State/Zip _____

Sex_____ Birthday _____

Hm. Phone _____Wk. Phone _____

How did you learn of us?

1. ☐ Friend _____   5. ☐ Lecture

2. ☐ Employee _____   6. ☐ Direct Mail

3. ☐ Newspaper   7. ☐ Welcome Basket

4. ☐ Location/Sign   8. ☐ Yellow Pages

Your Occupation?

1. ☐ Homemaker   6. ☐ Child (under 16)

2. ☐ Clerical   7. ☐ Student

3. ☐ Professional   8. ☐ Sr. Citizen

4. ☐ Technical   9. ☐ Self-Employed

5. ☐ Management   10. ☐ Sales

How often have you visited a salon in the past?

☐ Weekly

☐ Every 4 to 6 weeks

☐ Every 3 to 4 months

☐ Other _____

Have you ever had a permanent wave? _____

   Within the last year? _____

Have you ever had a hair color service? _____

   Within the last year? _____

What salon services do you usually require?

☐ Hair Analysis   ☐ Shampoo & Style   ☐ Recondition

☐ Haircut   ☐ Styling   ☐ Perm

☐ Hair Relaxing   ☐ Color   ☐ Bleach

☐ Pedicure   ☐ Sculptured Nails   ☐ Manicure

☐ Waxing   ☐ Eyebrow Arch   ☐ Electrolysis

Please list brand name of hair products you are using at home:

Shampoo _____

Conditioner or Rinse _____

Hair Spray _____

Styling Lotion _____

How often do you shampoo your hair? Every _____ days.

Which of these products are you using at home?

☐ Brush ☐ Hot Comb ☐ Blow Dryer ☐ Curling Iron

☐ Hot Rollers ☐ Comb ☐ Towel Dry

☐ Other _____

Are you taking any medication?_____

If so, please describe _____

_____

Do you have any allergies?_____

If so, please describe_____

_____

Why did you leave your last hairdresser? _____

_____

_____

_____

_____

_____

The above client information is strictly confidential, used solely for evaluation purposes within the salon.

ends of her hair will be chemically processed. It is common for a client to have more than one perm on their hair and not be aware of it. If the answer to this question is yes, ask the client how many perms she has had within the past year.

Monique: *Joan, how many perms have you had within the past year?*

Joan: *I had a perm two months ago. I had to go back because it didn't take the first time.*

Monique: *How long before that did you get a perm?*

Joan: *I always got perms regularly—every three months. My hair has no body.*

Monique: *Does your hair have body right after your perm?*

Joan: *Yes, for about six weeks—then it's gone. Flat and limp again. I have the worst hair of anyone I know.*

Question: *Have you ever had a color service? Within the past year?* (Joan answered yes to both questions.)

Monique: *Joan, from the looks of your new growth, you had color just a few weeks ago. Is that right?*

Joan: *Yes, I had color exactly two weeks ago. I have worn the same color for years, ever since I started to turn gray. What do you think of it? Does it need to be changed?*

Monique: *I think your color is great. Just enough gold in it to warm your skin. I think you should keep it. Do you have it done every month?*

Joan: *Every five weeks when I get my haircut.*

Question: *What salon services do you usually require?*

According to Joan's questionnaire, she has used a variety of salon services in the past. Monique will use Joan's responses to sell additional services today and secure them for future appointments.

Monique: *Joan, we have a very talented nail technician here. Her name is Carolyn and she does great pedicures and manicures. Do you usually get your pedicure and manicure on the same day as your color and cut?*

Joan: *Yes, I like to do that. I only get a pedicure every other time, though.*

Monique: *Today you are only scheduled for a haircut and style. Would you like me to see if Carolyn has time to do your nails when we finish your cut?*

Joan: *That would be great. I didn't even think about it when I scheduled my appointment with you.*

Monique: *Would you also like to have your brows arched while you are here?*

Joan: *No, not today. I have to go to lunch right after and I don't want to take the chance that my eyes might look red.*

Question: *Please list the brand name of the products you use at home.*

Joan uses all professional products on her hair. After Monique has analyzed Joan's hair and assessed her needs, she will talk to Joan about her hair products.

Question: *How often do you shampoo your hair?*

Joan shampoos her hair every other day. Monique will use this question and the following one as an opening to find out how much time Joan spends on her hair.

Question: *What styling tools are you using at home?*

Joan uses a blow dryer and curling iron on her hair.

Monique: *How much time do you want to spend on your hair when you style it?*

Joan: *It really takes me way too much time to do my hair. I think I spend forty-five minutes every time I wash it. I think that would be OK if my hair was long and thick. But this fine, thin hair shouldn't take more than twenty or thirty minutes. Don't you think?*

Monique: *You're right, Joan. It shouldn't take that long. Especially since your hair would probably dry in ten minutes. We'll work on a style that is easier, and I'll teach you some styling shortcuts that might help you out.*

Joan: *That sounds great, Monique. If you can make this hair easier for me, I'll be a client for life.*

Question: *Are you taking any medications? Do you have any allergies?*

Medications can interfere with chemical processing and be indications of clients' health problems. Joan isn't taking medications, but she has experienced allergic reactions to some skin care products.

Question: *Why did you leave your last hairdresser?*

Joan left her last hairdresser because Joan needed a change. Monique must find out if Joan's motivation to change stylists was more than because her stylist didn't suggest a change in hairstyle.

Monique: *You said that you needed a change. Did you just feel like you needed to get a new style?*

Joan: *Yes. My last stylist was really a nice girl, but she didn't know what to do with this fine hair. I kept asking for something new, but she didn't have any ideas.*

The Cutting and Styling Consultation

After the general consultation using the questionnaire, conduct a more specific consultation concerning the services that are being done today. If your client is new, you will have consulted with her using the client information form. If she is a returning client, you will have a different set of questions to ask (like the one's

Monique is using). For now we will return to Monique and her client Joan.

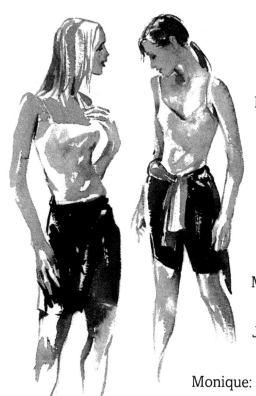

Monique: *Joan, tell me about some specific problems you are having with your hair right now.*

Joan: *Well, it's much too long. I haven't had it cut for seven weeks. It always goes flat on top. It's very straight—and limp. It's baby fine, has static in the winter, and flies straight up in the air. It lays down when I condition it, but it's totally flat an hour after I shampoo it. If you can fix all that, you are truly a miracle worker.*

Monique: *I don't think I'm a miracle worker; however, I'm sure we can fix some of your problems. Joan, have you ever had a haircut that was absolutely manageable?*

Joan: *Yes, I did. A few years ago I was on vacation in Paris. I went to a hairdresser and he cut my hair very short. I hated it at first, but about two months later it turned into a great haircut. My husband hated it, though. He doesn't like my hair short.*

Monique: *Describe that haircut to me. How long was it on top when you really liked it?*

Joan: *It was just long enough to get my curling iron around it and it didn't have a perm.*

Monique: *What if I cut your hair short on top and let it get gradually longer toward the back? It could be as long in the back as it is now. That should satisfy your husband's need to have some length on your hair and will allow your hair to have some lift on top. I don't think you'll need your hair permed for this style.*

Joan: *Sounds good to me. Do you have a picture that is similar to what you are talking about?*

Monique: *Yes, I know there are several styling books with similar cuts. I'll get some for you.*

Joan (after she has seen a few photos of similar styles): *I think you're right, Monique. Go ahead and cut it in the style you want.*

Monique: *Great, Joan. I know you'll like it.*

When Monique is finished with Joan's haircut, she will write notes on the questionnaire so she remembers what she and Joan discussed.

Clients return because they were happy with the last services they received. Consulting with return clients requires a slightly different approach. For the client's return visit, it is helpful to have the original questionnaire to use for reference. Let's join Marc, whose next client is Bob Sacks (who is returning for his fourth haircut). Marc has already looked over his previous notes on the questionnaire, greeted Bob, and escorted him to the styling chair.

Marc: *How was your last haircut, Bob?*

Bob: *It was good, Marc. I liked the way it grew out. In fact, I would like it to be just a little longer this time. And don't forget about my receding hairline.*

Marc: *Yes. I remember that you like to have your part higher than the natural split and long enough to cover both temples. Right?*

Bob: *That's right.*

Marc: *You also like to be shampooed after your cut to remove all the loose hairs.*

Bob: *That's what I like about this place. You people are always on top of things.*

For the client's return visit, it is helpful to have the original questionnaire to use for reference.

In another area of the salon, John is consulting with a return client who is not as pleased as Marc's client.

Eva: *John, the haircut you did last time was terrible. The first two cuts you did for me were wonderful What happened last time?*

John: *Eva, tell me specifically what was wrong with your cut.*

Eva: *Well, for one thing, the bangs were too short. I like them the length they are right now. The top stood up in the center and the sides went flat. My head was pointed like a football.*

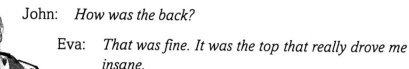

John: *How was the back?*

Eva: *That was fine. It was the top that really drove me insane.*

John: *It looks like I cut the top too short.*

Eva: *Yeah, probably, because you left me to take two phone calls while you were cutting my hair.*

John: *Oh, yes. That was the day my dog was having surgery. I'm sorry that I was distracted from your haircut. I won't let that happen again.*

Eva: *How is your dog, anyway?*

John: *She is just fine now. Let me review your haircut again before I start cutting.*

Simply knowing that they will have an opportunity to discuss problems with their hair during a consultation will bring even unhappy clients back to your salon. You will get a second chance because clients know you'll take the time to listen.

Reevaluating Clients

Reevaluate your clients regularly. The primary reason that clients leave their hairdresser is because the hairdresser didn't suggest change. It doesn't matter if your client has been with you for two visits or two hundred: Each client deserves a consultation every time and a total reevaluation every year. Clients change as they age and as their life situation changes. Hair becomes more gray and does not color the same as before. Texture can change. Curly hair gets straighter and straight hair can get wavy. Hair thins with illnesses and medications. Although the changes are gradual, they are changes nonetheless and must be recognized and dealt with.

Carl's next client is Margaret, who has been coming to Sensations Salon for fifteen years. Today, since Carl has a few extra minutes in his schedule, he will devote extra time to Margaret's color. He has noticed that recently her color has lost some shine and looks a little lifeless. Carl greets Margaret and begins to examine her hair.

Carl: *Hello, Margaret, how are the grandchildren doing? Have they visited lately?*

Margaret: *Yes, they were here last weekend. I kept them while my son and daughter-in-law were away for a few days. They were certainly a handful.*

Carl: *Margaret, I have a little extra time today so I'd like to talk to you about your haircolor. Does it seem more drab than it used to be?*

Margaret: *Now that you mention it, yes it does. I have noticed that it looks lighter, too. Did you change the color?*

Carl: *No. I think your hair is changing and we need to adjust your color.*

Margaret: *You mean I'm getting more gray. You don't have to be so diplomatic about it, Carl. I'll be fifty this year, so I guess it's OK to have some gray hair.*

Carl: *The gray hair colors differently than your natural ash blonde. I would like to keep it in the lighter shade and add a little warmth to the color. How does that sound?*

Margaret: *You don't mean my hair will be gold, do you?*

Carl: *No, Margaret, it will be a soft warm blonde. The slightly warmer tone will go better with your skin tone, too.*

Margaret: *OK, Carl. Let's try it.*

Reevaluate your clients regularly. Each client deserves a consultation every time and a total reevaluation every year.

Some Questions to Ask a Returning Client

How did your last haircut work out for you?

Did you have any problem areas?

Let me review how your hair was cut last time.

Are you looking for a change in style or simply a maintenance cut?

Would you like to see some alternate ways of finishing this style?

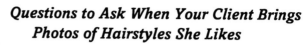

Questions to Ask When Your Client Brings Photos of Hairstyles She Likes

What do you like about the pictures or about that particular style in the picture? Do you like the top, front, sides, or bang area? (Sometimes clients only like one particular area of a style.)

Do you like the length? (Show the client what that length would look like on her.)

What do you dislike about the hairstyle in the picture? (It is possible that the very area of the style that you think makes that style distinctive is the same part the client hates.)

Questions to Ask Yourself When a Client Brings a Photo of a Hairstyle

Does the client have a similar face shape and hair texture as the model in the picture? (If the face shape and texture are different, it will be difficult to reproduce the look.)

Will she need a perm to do the new style?

How much time will be required to do the new style? Will it be complicated?

Be sure to comb and clip the client's hair into a similar shape to see if she likes it.

The Color Consultation

Because color changes, it is important to have color consultations every time clients have a color service. Repeating the same color service on clients year after year without recognizing changes in the client's hair or the shifts in fashion trends will lose clients. A color technician who is constantly learning new techniques and delivers quality service can attract more loyalty from clients than any other salon professional.

Because words describing color are all relative, photos of

often occurs between professionals and clients. To a client, strawberry blonde color can be anything from golden blonde to light auburn. The word *ash* to a professional can signify "drab" but to a client it can mean "soft." Even a manufacturer's color chart doesn't communicate as well as a photograph, in which the client can see the color on a person.

Some important information you should get and give during the color consultation is as follows:

Has the client had any history of sensitivity to color services?

Has the client ever had any kind of color, including rinses, wash-in color, semipermanent color, henna, etc.? Was it done in a salon or at home?

What is the purpose of the color service? Is it to cover gray, to enhance a style, to brighten the natural color, or to create a new look?

Does the client like monotone colors, highlighting color, or multicolor? (Again, this is where photos clarify statements.)

Inform the client about how often the color should be done to keep it looking good and then find out if the client is able to commit to that.

Educate the client about the special products required for color-treated hair.

Find out if the client is planning to perm his or her hair.

Because words describing color are all relative, photos of color are an excellent way to bridge the communication gap that often occurs between professionals and clients.

Carl is the salon's color and perm technician. Today he is running a little behind schedule. He is consulting with a new client, Jenna Gray, when his next client, Rosalyn, arrives for her monthly touch-up. Carl summons Robert, his assistant, to help. Carl excuses himself from Jenna while he speaks to Robert.

Carl: *Robert, please have Rosalyn change into a gown and prepare her for color.*

Robert: *Do you want me to go ahead and apply it for you?*

Carl: *Probably, but I want to talk to her first.*
(Robert escorts Rosalyn to the color and perm area of the salon, where Carl is speaking to Jenna.)

Carl: *Jenna, I don't want to rush through your color consulta-*

tion. We need to talk a while longer before I'm satisfied that we are on the same wavelength. Would you mind if I take a minute to get Robert started on my next client?

Jenna: *Sure, go ahead. Your receptionist told me to plan on being here a few hours today since it's my first time here.*

Carl : *Thank you, Jenna. I'll just be a few minutes. Robert will refill your coffee if you are ready.*

Jenna: *No thanks, I'm fine. I have a book to read.*
(Carl turns to Rosalyn.)

Carl: *How are you, Rosalyn? Looks like you just got back from a sunny vacation.*

Rosalyn: *I had a wonderful vacation in Hawaii.*

Carl: *You didn't tell me you were going to Hawaii.*

Rosalyn: *I didn't know. It was my husband's anniversary gift to me. I don't know how he pulled it off but it was certainly a surprise. He even made arrangements with my boss to have time off.*

Carl: *He sounds like a perfect husband to me. And you got a beautiful tan—but I see that your haircolor is more faded than usual and the ends feel really dry. We'll need to do a treatment before your color. How about if we leave the ends a little lighter until your tan fades?*

Rosalyn: *I'll leave it up to you, Carl. You always do a good job.*

Carl: *Robert will give your hair a treatment, I'll get your color prepared and then Robert will apply it for you, OK? I'll get a chance to talk to you later, and maybe you can tell me all about Hawaii.*

Rosalyn: *Carl, be sure Robert knows about my sensitive scalp!*

Robert: *Don't worry, Rosalyn, Carl already told me to be very gentle with your scalp. Come with me and I'll get you shampooed first.*
(Carl returns to Jenna, his new client.)

Carl: *OK, Jenna. Let's talk about your haircolor. You say you would like your hair highlighted with blondes?*

Jenna: *I want a lot of blonde. It would be great to have my hair blonde like it was a few years a go, before I had children.*

Carl: *Is the color on your ends about the shade you would like to have?*

Jenna: *Yes, it is. Can you make it that color all over?*

Carl: *You mean highlight it with that color?*

Jenna: *Yes, but I want a lot of it.*

Carl: *How would you feel about natural-looking highlights all over with a few bolder streaks around your face?*

Jenna: *That sounds terrific. I didn't think about doing streaks.*

Carl: *Jenna, I want to design this color around your style. Are you going to keep your hair in this style or are you going to change it?*

Jenna: *I don't think I want to change it yet, but I have been toying with the idea of getting the back cut shorter. Nothing drastic, though.*

Carl: *I have a photo of the look I would like to do on you* (shows her the photo). *Do you like it?*

Jenna: *When you said bold, you meant bold, didn't you. I don't think I want streaks like that.*

Carl: *How about if they aren't so wide? About half that size would be good on you.*

Jenna: *I do like the shade of blonde in the photo—but I don't know about streaks . . . Oh well, go ahead, let's do it.*

The Perm Consultation

A preshampoo consultation is more important when perming clients' hair than before almost any other service. Ask questions to find out how much old perm is still on the client's hair and what tools she used to style her hair. Was it air dried, smoothed out with a styling brush, or ironed? Thoroughly analyze the client's hair texture, pliability, and porosity before shampooing and again after.

Some important information you should get and give during the perm consultation is as follows:

Did you like your last perm?

Have you ever experienced problems with a perm?

How long do your perms usually last?

Have you ever experienced sensitivities to perm solution?

How long since your last color service?

Do you have hard or soft water at home?

What tools will you use to finish your hair?

After the hair has been shampooed, find out the client's history of permanent waving on her hair.

<table>
<tr><td>Jennifer:</td><td>I see on your questionnaire that you have had perms before. When did you have your last perm?</td></tr>
<tr><td>Kathy:</td><td>I don't think there is any perm left in my hair. It's been four months and it's really straight now.</td></tr>
<tr><td>Jennifer:</td><td>Your hair is about shoulder length, so all but about 2 inches of new growth is chemically treated hair. How long before that did you have a perm?</td></tr>
<tr><td>Kathy:</td><td>Probably four months. I usually get my hair permed every four months.</td></tr>
<tr><td>Jennifer:</td><td>That means that the ends of your hair have had at least three perms on them. Do you have difficulty getting the ends of your hair to curl?</td></tr>
<tr><td>Kathy:</td><td>Yes, it curls fine up here (pointing to the mid-shaft of her hair). But the ends always go limp. My hair is so straight I just have to have a perm. I don't really want to have short hair, but I don't know what else to do with it.</td></tr>
<tr><td>Jennifer:</td><td>Well, Kathy, your hair has been through too much perming. It only grows about half an inch a month, so it has only grown out 2 inches when you get your four-month perm. Can you see that when your hair is 14 inches long and it has had a perm every 2 inches, the ends of your hair have multiple processes? There are several things we can do. First of all, I think if you get it cut just a few inches, you</td></tr>
</table>

A preshampoo consultation is more important when perming clients' hair than before almost any other service.

could get rid of the worst of the damaged hair. Another option is to have a series of treatments.

Kathy: *Jennifer, I use all the best products on my hair. I use conditioner every time I shampoo. I even use this oil on the ends to make my hair shine.*

Jennifer: *What I am recommending is a series of salon treatments. They will accomplish much more than a conditioner you use at home.*

Kathy: *Does that mean I can get another perm and not have to get my hair cut?*

Jennifer: *The treatments should allow you to save more length; however, I'm sure that even with treating your hair you will have to have some cut. The treatments in combination with a specialized wrapping method and perm for your type of hair will allow us to perm your hair safely.*

Kathy: *Jennifer, you are a lifesaver. I'm so glad I found you.*

The Nail Consultation

Too often consultations with nail clients happen after there is a problem. Allergic reactions to nail chemicals, skin that is damaged easily, and skin that is prone to infection are all conditions that nail techs should be aware of before any nail service. Sensations Salon uses an additional client questionnaire for nail clients to be sure that the nail tech learns all about the client's nails before the service.

Carolyn, our nail technician, uses the nail questionnaire to consult with her new client.

Carolyn: *Hello, Joan, it's nice to meet you. I am Carolyn, your nail technician. Sit down right here at the table.*

Nail Questionnaire

Name _____ Date _____

Address _____ Day Phone _____

City/State/Zip _____

1. How did you hear about our nail services?
   - ☐ Friend _____ ☐ Employee _____
   - ☐ Advertising _____ ☐ Other _____

2. What is your occupation? _____

3. Do you have any of the following health problems? Check all that apply.
   - ☐ Diabetes   ☐ Hormonal problems
   - ☐ High/low blood pressure   ☐ Pregnancy
   - ☐ Allergies   ☐ Recent surgery
   - Please list _____

4. Which nail services have you used in the past?
   - ☐ Manicure   ☐ Cooling foot masque
   - ☐ French manicure   ☐ Gel nails
   - ☐ Paraffin treatment   ☐ Nail tips
   - ☐ AHA hand treatment   ☐ Sculptured nails
   - ☐ Pedicure   ☐ Fiberglass nails
   - ☐ Paraffin foot treatment ☐ Nail art
   - ☐ AHA foot treatment   ☐ Hand and arm massage
   - ☐ Reflexology

5. Have you ever been treated by a physician for a nail disorder? _____

6. Have you ever had any of the following nail disorders?
   - ☐ Ridged nails   ☐ Brittle nails
   - ☐ White spots on nails   ☐ Thick nails
   - ☐ Bitten nails   ☐ Ingrown nails
   - ☐ Hangnails   ☐ Infection of nail or surrounding tissue
   - ☐ Thin nails   ☐ Fungus
   - ☐ Bruised nails

7. Have you ever experienced an allergic reaction to a nail product or any ingredients found in nail-products? _____

   If so, please describe _____

The above client information is strictly confidential and is used only for evaluation purposes in the salon.

Joan: *It's nice to meet you too, Carolyn. I'm glad you had time for me today.*

Carolyn: *I see Monique recommended you. Did she cut your hair today? It looks wonderful.*

Joan: *Yes, thank you. I like it too.*

Carolyn: *Let me look at your hands. On your questionnaire you say that you had gel nails in the past. You don't have them now. Did you have problems with them?*

Joan: *No. I only had them put on for a special occasion. I kept them a month and then had them removed.*

Carolyn: *Today you need a manicure, right?*

Joan: *Well, I need a whole lot more than that, but what I want today is just a manicure.*

Carolyn: *OK. Your hands seem a little dry. Would you also like to have a paraffin treatment?*

Joan: *If you have time, go ahead.*

Carolyn: *Joan, have you ever had any problems with your hands during a manicure, such as sensitive cuticles?*

Joan: *No, I haven't. My hands are pretty tough. You can push hard on my cuticles and it doesn't hurt.*

Carolyn: *Would you like your rings cleaned while I do your manicure?*

Joan: *Yes, that would be wonderful.*

Carolyn: *I see on your questionnaire that you have been treated for nail disorders. Can you tell me about it?*

Joan: *It was my toenails. Once I had an ingrown toenail that had to be removed, and another time I had a fungus under my toenail. The doctor said I probably picked it up while I was on vacation in South America. I got a pedicure at a salon down there. Don't worry, though, that was three years ago.*

Carolyn: *Are you about ready to schedule another pedicure?*

Joan: *Yes, I have them regularly. I love getting pedicures.*

Carolyn: *Take a look at the nail colors on the shelf beside you and see which one you would like today. There is a color called Peach Whip that I think would go well with your skin.*

Consultation for Artificial Nails

Carolyn: *Hello, Jessica, it's nice to meet you. My name is Carolyn and I'm your nail technician today. I see that you want artificial nails but aren't quite sure which kind you want. Is that right?*

Jessica: *Yes. I'd like to know what my options are.*

Carolyn: *Sit down and we'll talk for a few minutes while I prepare your nails. Your hands are beautiful. You are going to love having long nails.*

Jessica: *I don't want them very long because I'm getting married in about six weeks and I want my nails to look good in the pictures.*

Carolyn: *Congratulations, Jessica! Do you plan on keeping your artificial nails after the wedding?*

Jessica: *Maybe. I'm in sales and it would be nice to have my hands look good all the time.*

Carolyn: *OK. Let's go over the different types of nails. First, acrylic nails are also called sculptured nails because a liquid and powder are mixed together into a paste and then sculpted onto your nail with a brush. Acrylic nails are by far the hardest type of nails. If you like long nails or if you have weak natural nails, you would do well with acrylics. Maintenance with acrylics should be every two weeks. Here is a current price list that you can refer to as we talk.*

Jessica: *My natural nails must be weak since I can't seem to grow them.*

Carolyn: *That isn't necessarily true. Maybe you can't grow them because of the way you use them. Many people abuse their nails without even realizing it. Like using them to pry things or not wearing gloves in harsh detergents or when gardening.*

Jessica: *You're right. I'm guilty of all those things.*

Carolyn: *Your nails look strong to me. Maybe you would like to have gel nails. Gels can be used with tips for added length or as an overlay on your natural nail. Gels are flexible and very natural looking. However, due to their flexibility, they can break more easily at the stress point. That's right here where the free edge meets the nail bed. Gels need to be rebalanced every three weeks.*

Jessica: *I guess I should get gels nails, shouldn't I?*

Carolyn: *Maybe, but first we have to talk about your hobbies. How active are you?*

Jessica: *I like to work out at the health club, and my fiancé and I play tennis once or twice a week. I think that could damage my nails. Maybe I should get acrylics.*

Carolyn: *I think so. Acrylic it is. I have an information sheet for you that tells you all about acrylic nails and how to care for them at home. In addition, all our acrylic nail clients get a Hand and Nail Maintenance Kit to take home. I'll show you how to use it when we are finished with your nails.*

Jessica: *What a nice thing to do. I'm really excited to get my nails!*

The Pedicure Consultation

Carolyn uses the same questionnaire for all nail care services, including pedicures. In addition, she will ask the client questions about sensitivity to heat or cold, tenderness or ticklishness, and foot or skin problems. When she has a client who is new to pedicuring, she will briefly explain the procedure so that the client isn't taken by surprise by any of the manipulations.

Carolyn's next client is a male client in his early fifties. This is his first pedicure.

YOUR SCULPTURED NAILS
DO'S AND DON'TS

DO

Take off polish before your appointments to decrease your time in the salon.

Have regular maintenance rebalancing. Recommended maintenance is two weeks for acrylics and three weeks for gel nails.

Use only products recommended by your nail technician.

Always wear gloves when using cleaning products or any other chemicals that can damage nails.

Call if you have any questions.

DON'T

NEVER GLUE A WET OR NON-DISINFECTED NAIL ONTO YOUR NAIL BED. Glue and disinfectant are included in your nail maintenance kit.

NEVER pry, bite, or pull artificial nails to remove them. We can use special chemicals to remove them with little damage to your nail bed.

Since nails absorb water like a sponge, avoid water for at least an hour before your appointment time. Saturation includes bathing, showering, and washing dishes.

Do not expose nails to extreme heat at any time on the day of your appointment. Saunas and extreme hot water are in this category. Tanning will not affect your nails.

Never use baby oil or any products with lanolin or mineral oil, which will promote lifting.

Carolyn: *Hello, Mr. Brown. My name is Carolyn and I will be doing your pedicure today. This is your first pedicure, isn't it?*

Mr. Brown: *Please call me Mike, Carolyn. This is the first time I've had a pedicure. My wife made the appointment for me because I am always complaining about what a hassle it is to cut my toenails. She says that you told her that if I had them cut properly I wouldn't have as much trouble with ingrown nails.*

Carolyn: *Your wife is Nancy, right? I just love doing her nails. Let's begin by soaking your feet in the foot bath. There, how is that? Is the water warm enough?*

Mike: *That feels great. You probably don't often work on feet as big and ugly as mine, do you?*

Carolyn: *Mike, everybody thinks their feet are ugly. Most people neglect their feet until they start to have problems with them—you know, wearing shoes that don't exactly fit. I think women tend to do that more than men, but I see you have corns and calluses too. Are you on your feet a lot at work?*

Nail techs can use the same questionnaire for all nail care services including pedicures.

Mike: *Yes, I'm a hospital administrator. It sounds like a job where I would sit all day, but it seems like I am always walking the corridors.*

Carolyn: *Today I'll show you the proper length and shape for your toenails. Since it looks like you have a tendency to have ingrown nails, you should get pedicures every five weeks. If you do that, I can work on these calluses and make sure you don't get ingrown nails again. How does that sound?*

Mike: *It sounds a whole lot easier than trying to do it myself.*

Carolyn: *Wonderful. After a few pedicures, you won't recognize your own feet.*

Mike: *Carolyn, my wife, said that you also do reflexology. Can you tell me a little bit about it?*

The Reflexology Consultation

Carolyn: *Reflexology is a science that deals with the principle that there are reflex areas in the feet and hands which correspond to all of the glands, organs, and parts of the body. It is a unique method where I use my thumbs and forefingers to manipulate these reflex areas. You can see where they are in this diagram.*

Mike: *I've seen a picture in a magazine of the foot and all the organs drawn on the bottom. It looked very interesting, but I'm very ticklish.*

Carolyn: *I understand. However, I don't skim lightly on the skin. I use some pressure, and most people who are ticklish respond very well. It shouldn't hurt, and using pressure reduces ticklishness. If there is anyplace I work that is sensitive, I'll reduce the pressure.*

Mike: *Do people do this just because it feels good?*

Carolyn: *It can be very relaxing, but there are many benefits to reflexology. It relieves stress, and you know that many diseases and illness come from stress. It improves circulation and nerve responses, and it can ease muscle contraction in all your glands and organs.*

Mike: *Sounds like something I need, Carolyn. Do you have time for reflexology today?*

Carolyn: *Yes, I think I do. It's a wonderful service to have after a pedicure.*

Mike: *What are you doing?*

Carolyn: *I'm taking a closer look at those calluses. Sometimes they cause pressure on reflexes. You know the old saying "When your feet hurt, everything hurts?" Doesn't that make sense now that you've seen my reflexology diagram?*

Mike: *It sure does. I'm really looking forward to this.*

Reflexology is a science that deals with the principle that there are reflex areas in the feet and hands which correspond to all of the glands, organs, and parts of the body.

Margo: Good afternoon. You must be Jackie Collier.

Jackie: Yes, I'm here for a facial.

Margo: You have a one o'clock appointment with Suzanne. Would you please fill out this questionnaire for her? As soon as you are finished, I will have an assistant take you to the facial area.

(Jackie returns the completed questionnaire to Margo and is escorted to the salon's facial area.)

Suzanne: Here is a gown for you. Change into it and sit in the facial chair. I'll be right back. There are clothing hooks on the door.

Suzanne   (returns a few minutes later): You can have your choice of music during your facial. Do you like classical, nature sounds, soft jazz, or new age music? Which would you like?

Jackie: I usually like classical music. Is that all right with you?

Suzanne: Sure, that will be fine. Just lie down there nice and comfortable and we'll get started. Is this your first facial?

Jackie: No, but it's the first time I have had a facial here.

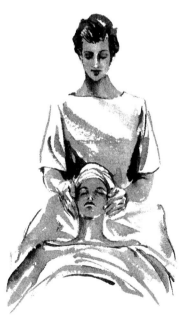

Suzanne: Well, since it's your first time here, I'll have to do a skin analysis before I start your facial. First I'll clean your face and then I'll turn this magnifying light on and examine your skin. You don't have to do anything except answer a few questions. I see on your questionnaire that you wear contact lenses. Would you like to remove them?

Jackie: No. My eyes aren't sensitive at all, and I've never had a problem wearing them and getting facials in the past.

(Suzanne cleans Jackie's face and examines it through the magnifying lamp.)

Skin Care Information

Name _____ Date _____

Address _____ Day Phone _____

City/State/Zip _____

1. How did you hear about our skin and body care services?
   - ☐ Friend _____ ☐ Employee _____
   - ☐ Family _____ ☐ Other _____
   - ☐ Advertising _____

2. Which of the following services have you used in the past?
   - ☐ Massotherapy   ☐ Treatment facial
   - ☐ Herbal body polish ☐ Oily skin facial
   - ☐ European facial   ☐ AHA facial
   - ☐ Paraffin facial   ☐ Herbology facial

3. Do you have any of the following health problems? Check all that apply.
   - ☐ Diabetes   ☐ Hormonal Problems
   - ☐ High/low blood pressure ☐ Sinus Problems
   - ☐ Malfunctioning Thyroid ☐ Skin Cancer
   - ☐ Allergies _____

Have you had recent surgery?	Y	N
If so, what _____		
Are you or do you:		
Pregnant	Y	N
Take medications	Y	N
Have implants	Y	N
Have pacemaker	Y	N
Wear contact lenses	Y	N
Use retin-A	Y	N
Under a lot of stress	Y	N
Exposed to pollution	Y	N

What improvements would you like to see in your skin? _____
_____

Are you under or have you had medical care for skin problems?
If so, please describe.

_____
_____

Have you ever had a negative reaction to a skin care product?

Which product _____

Cleanser _____

Moisturizer _____

Night creme _____

Eye creme _____

Mask _____

Margo	(on the phone): *Good afternoon, Sensations Salon. This is Margo. May I help you?*
Kimberly:	*Do you do leg waxing?*
Margo:	*Yes, we do. May I schedule an appointment for you?*
Kimberly:	*I think so. I've never had it done before. Can I get an appointment right away?*
Margo:	*Could I have your name, please?*
Kimberly:	*This is Kimberly Kantor.*
Margo:	*Hi, Kimberly. Before you schedule an appointment, you need to know that you have to let your hair grow about four weeks in order to get good results.*
Kimberly:	*Yes. I already know that. You see, I have this friend who lives in Washington who has been trying to get me to wax my legs for a long time. She has hers done regularly and says that once I do it I'll never go back to shaving. So I let my hair grow and now I think it's long enough to wax. Do you have an opening today?*
Margo:	*You are in luck, Kimberly. Suzanne just had a facial cancel. You can have an appointment at three o'clock.*
Kimberly:	*Great. I'll be there.*

At three o'clock, Suzanne is examining Kimberly's hair and skin and consulting about leg waxing.

Suzanne:	*Your hair is dark and fairly coarse. We'll get good results today; however, your hair grows in several stages. Right now, even though you haven't shaved for four weeks, some of the hairs are just breaking through the skin and will be too short for today's procedure.*
Kimberly:	*You mean I'll still have stubble in a few days?*

Suzanne:	Yes. Until I've waxed your legs three or four times, about once a month, you may still experience some stubble. After that, however, the hair gets sort of wimpy. It seems to grow in a finer texture and it's lighter and softer. You won't notice the growth as much as you do now.
Kimberly:	Oh, yeah, my friend Melanie told me that. She also said it didn't hurt a bit. I just can't believe that.
Suzanne:	Well, whether it hurts or not depends on the person. Some people are more sensitive than others. And there are some areas of the body that will tingle a little. Today we'll be working on a lot of coarse hair so it may sting a little more. In the future, when the hair becomes finer and softer it will be much easier to remove. Most people say it feels like taking a tape bandage off your skin.
Kimberly:	I usually have a high tolerance for discomfort, so I don't think this will bother me too much.
Suzanne:	There are other benefits to leg waxing besides the hair removal. Your skin will be smoother. You see, the waxing process also exfoliates the skin, so you won't have any of this dry flaky skin on your legs for a while. It also stimulates circulation in your legs.
Kimberly:	That sounds great. I always seem to have dry skin on my legs.
Suzanne:	There are a few other questions I need to ask you. Have you ever had any allergies, particularly skin allergies?
Kimberly:	I don't think so.
Suzanne:	Have you ever had a negative reaction to any skin product?
Kimberly:	Yes, but that was a facial mask that made me break out.
Suzanne:	Is your skin sensitive?
Kimberly:	Yes, I think it is. It turns red easily, but it doesn't hurt and the redness goes away quickly.
Suzanne:	Since this is your first time, Kimberly, I'm going to remove one strip on your legs and then wait about five minutes to see if there is any sensitivity. OK?
Kimberly:	Sounds good to me.

1. Consulting is the process of discovery in which the stylist observes, studies, and detects what the client needs.

2. Consulting's purpose is also to reveal problems that clients might not be aware of, such as hair breakage, product build-up, dry, frizzy hair, or mismatched color.

3. A preshampoo consultation allows clients to be more comfortable talking to stylists. When clients are comfortable, it is easier for them to explain what they want.

4. During a shampoo consultation with clients, you find out if they like a firm or gentle massage, warm or cool water, and one or two shampoos and whether or not they have sensitive scalps.

5. Using a client questionnaire will enhance consultations. It saves stylists and technicians time, answers many pertinent questions, and gives the stylist openings for additional questions that could improve the overall results of the client's service.

6. After the general consultation with the questionnaire, conduct a more specific consultation concerning the services that are being done for the client today.

7. Consulting with return clients requires a slightly different approach. For the client's return visit, it is helpful to refer to the original questionnaire.

8. Reevaluate your clients regularly. The primary reason that clients leave their hairdresser is that the hairdresser didn't suggest change. It doesn't matter if your client has been with you for two visits or two hundred: Each client deserves a consultation every time and a total reevaluation every year.

9. Because color changes, it is important to have color consultations every time clients have a color service. Repeating the same color service on clients year after year without recognizing changes in the client's hair or the shifts in fashion trends will lose clients.

10. A preshampoo consultation is more important when perming clients' hair than before almost any other service. Ask questions to find out how much old perm is still on the client's hair and what tools she used to style her hair.

11. Too often consultations with nail clients happen after there is a problem. Allergic reactions to nail chemicals, skin that is damaged easily, and skin that is prone to infection are all conditions that nail techs should be aware of before any nail service.

12. Nail techs can use the same questionnaire for all nail care services, including pedicures. In addition, ask the client questions about sensitivity to heat or cold, tenderness or ticklishness, and foot or skin problems. For a client who is new to pedicuring, briefly explain the procedure so that the client isn't taken by surprise by any of the manipulations.

13. Reflexology is an easy add-on service for nail clients.

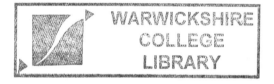

WARWICKSHIRE
COLLEGE
LIBRARY